NATURE—The Healer

NATURE—The Healer

by

JOHN T. RICHTER

Doctor of Chiropractic and Naturopathy
in Minnesota

As Edited by
HENRY W. SPLITTER, M. A.
(University of Wisconsin)

Published by
JOHN T. RICHTER
2844 Avenel Street
LOS ANGELES

1944

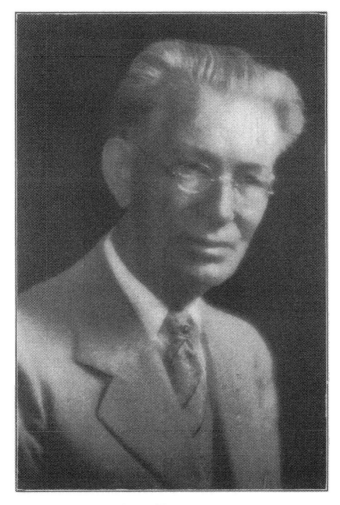

JOHN T. RICHTER

For Twenty-five Years Teacher of the Live Food Philosophy

We Dedicate This Book
to Humanity
Whom We Serve

INTRODUCTION

About two years ago Dr. Richter's wife, Mrs. Vera Richter, introduced me to the material which now comprises this book. A stenographer had been engaged to take down in shorthand the lectures which Dr. Richter was giving from time to time at the Richter live-food restaurants in Los Angeles. These lectures, together with the questions afterwards asked by the audience, were then typewritten. The style, of course, was the colloquial one suited to these informal lectures. The questions asked were impromptu; likewise the answers. Mrs. Richter thought it might be possible to work this material into a book suitable for the general reader, one who has no knowledge of technical medicine, but who would be interested in and profit by a discussion in simple language of Nature's method of healing. This naturally would involve a great deal of work—cutting down here, expanding there, rephrasing, re-arranging. Originally she had thought of doing this work herself, in spare time, but this proved unfeasible. As I had been a college instructor in English, moreover had myself lived for six years substantially according to the plan advocated by Dr. Richter, she thought I might be the man for the job. Hence I undertook this work and have been engaged on it at intervals ever since, with the aid of, during the last year, my wife, Clara Lipman Splitter.

As to the style, whenever possible the exact words of Dr. Richter have been preserved. The ideas throughout are his own, although I have expanded them considerably and have also myself added certain minor points which are, however, fully approved by Dr. Richter's experience. The question and answer form has been adopted because of its simplicity and directness.

Although the author is a Doctor of Chiropractic and Naturopathy, he has not practiced since coming to California. The management of his restaurants and educational work connected with the live-food movement have demanded his entire time.

HENRY W. SPLITTER.

Los Angeles, California,
October 1, 1936.

BIOGRAPHY

I have often been asked how I came to be a believer in live (uncooked) food, whether I was brought up in this manner, and if not, how long since I was con-verted to this new way of living. So perhaps a general outline of the facts may be illuminating and helpful to my readers.

My father was a country physician of the conventional medical type. He also owned a drug store in the little North Dakota town of Fargo in which I was raised. He wanted me to be a medical doctor, just as he was; but, as it happened, I had worked, as a young man, for nine years in his drug store, and had had plenty of experience in the compounding of inorganic drugs. I had observed their effects on my father's patients. He decided to send me to the Rush Medical College in Chicago, and he thought it strange when I showed no desire to fulfill his wishes.

However, I did go to Chicago, and soon got a position in a machine shop. Before the first winter was over, I had become acquainted with the so-called "movement cure," in which the general theory and practice of vegetarianism of the cooked-food type was incorporated. In my spare time I studied at the institute in which this health system was taught, finally graduated and received my diploma.

Since my father had been writing me for some time to come home, I decided I would. When I got there, I showed him my diploma. The first thing he said on seeing it was "quack," uttered emphatically and with disgust. Of course, nothing could have hurt me more than that. Yet I said, "Well, father, perhaps I will be good enough to drive your ponies." When I said that, I did not know what the final result of my taking over the coachman's job would be.

As we drove from place to place to see father's patients, he would tell me, perhaps, "We are going to see the French lady. She is suffering from rheumatism; has been in bed for three years; and is one of my charity patients. Of course, there is no cure for rheumatism; I just help her with liniment and make her comfortable." Again he would say, "There is Janet Smith. She has epilepsy—six to twelve spells a day, and she will always have it, poor girl. She is another charity patient." And so on. He had some fifteen or twenty patients, all with some supposedly incurable disease. One day an idea occurred to me. "Father, let me have all those cases you cannot cure, so that I will have some experience." He replied, "Very well, I shall ask the French lady if she is willing; also Janet Smith." These two cases were then turned over to me. After a short time, he gave me all the other "incurables" to care for as well.

I thought I would surprise father with the results which I had obtained. The French woman, under my care, was out of bed before two weeks were up, and in six months ventured to walk all the way to our office. Father had never seen her in street clothes. When she opened the office door, she saw father sitting behind his desk, and me at the library table. He did not recognize her by her appearance, but the moment she spoke he knew her. He greeted her and looked over toward me. She turned, came over to me, and kissed me; and father dropped his head. I walked out, leaving them there to converse together.

Two weeks later, father went out alone with the ponies, and saw someone who looked like Janet Smith going along unassisted. At first he could not trust his eyes, but he drove up closer and realized that they had not deceived him. He called out, "Are you on your way home? Get into the buggy and I'll take you there," motioning toward the seat. "You must tell me all about yourself." And she told him all that had happened. Father thought, "How amazing. These two people are well. I am going to look over the whole list of chronics and see if they're all well." Sure enough, he found they were all improved practically beyond recognition, some of them having even resumed their old trades. After he had made this trip of inspection, father came into the office, where he found me sitting. He walked up to me, slapped me heavily on the shoulder. I thought I had done something terrible for which he was about to reprove me. But he only said, "My son, I shall never call you 'quack' again." Then he told me about his experience.

Notice that all these cures were accomplished under the Battle Creek system of diet—cooked food vegetarianism, with a considerable amount of green vegetables and fruits. The results I had obtained were marvelous. How was it, then, that I finally decided the disease problem could be cured only by natural living, the most prominent feature of which being a diet consisting exclusively of uncooked fruits, nuts, and vegetables selected according to individual taste? I shall explain.

After having lived for fifteen years largely on a cooked-food diet (no meat, of course), I noticed that there was something physically wrong with me. My kidneys were not functioning properly. I seemed to lack recuperative energy. Although I did not feel ill enough to be in bed, I was constantly harassed by a "gone" feeling, lack of power to rebuild myself—in short, general lack of energy. Especially was this forced upon my attention once when I was called out into the country on a consultation. I was practicing independently at that time in Minneapolis. It was a long, hard trip—thirty miles over the prairies, and back to the city only at four in the morning. It was too late to have any real rest in bed, as I thought; therefore I simply waited around until it was time to have breakfast. Then I went to the office to get ready for business. The patients were already coming in, but I was so tired that every now and then I would find myself dozing over my work. I would shake myself, take a swallow of cold water, and rub cold water over my face. Yet in a moment or two I would again be nodding. I was nonplussed, not to say alarmed, at this lack of reserve energy. I became dizzy, too, at intervals. What was there in my system of living that was wrong? Had I not at least been eating correctly? That set me thinking.

It was not, however, until later that I became convinced it was really the food I had been eating which was at fault. This is how it came about: in a naturopathic magazine which had come to my hands, there was an article describing how a certain Dr. Lust had been invited by Dr. George Drews of Chicago to partake of an uncooked food dinner. It told of the many different varieties of food that were served, of how delicious they were. It said something, too, about raw pie. I thought, "How curious, unbaked pie!" I remembered how mother used to make hers. But this was raw pie. The whole idea took me by surprise. How can people live on uncooked food, I wondered, just as people today ask me the very same question.

I kept thinking about it, however, and finally decided to give this new diet a trial, to see if it would bring me that unlimited reserve of energy which I so ardently desired, as well as freedom from the more obvious diseases. Dr. Drew came to Minneapolis to teach me, as well as the class I had organized for him. Gradually, my health began improving, as the result of faithful adherence, one hundred per cent, to the prescribed diet. In six months such a change had been wrought in my body that it seemed logical to use the new system in my practice in order to observe how it would affect others. After a period of nine months, I realized that the nature of my bloodstream had been completely transformed. My blood, under tests, had previously shown too much acid present. Now it had become slightly alkaline, which is the normal state for one who is in first-rate health. We now know that cooked-food vegetarians, as well as meat eaters, alike suffer from too much acid in the bloodstream, as a rule. Nine months had been required in my case, but many others require only from three to six months. You can well suppose that I was very happy when I found my blood was sufficiently alkaline. What a mental relief and assurance to know that I was getting better at last! As to weight, when I first began, my 145 pounds dwindled away to 123. Many of my friends told me, as yours will undoubtedly tell you, that I had better quit before starving to death. Yet, realizing that my old, worn-out body cells had to be utterly eliminated before new cellular tissue could take their place, I remained faithful to my task. All the while, of course, even though seeming to be thin, I felt much better than I ever had before, and really did not care whether the scale index went up or down. Soon I redeemed that loss —redeemed every pound and a little additional.

For twenty-five years now I have lived according to this system. I was in the late forties when I started. Today, at seventy-two (I was born in 1864), I can do more work, can do it more accurately, than I could when I was thirty-five.

ABSCESSES

Q. What must one do to get rid of an abscess?

A. An abscess is a funnel of waste matter for the expelling of old broken-down mucous membrane. Almost every one alive has one in some form or other. Its principal cause is the eating of flesh food. Meat cannot digest in the human body, but merely decays and becomes waste matter that destroys everything it contacts. Eating of salt and all other indigestible and fixed elements will also help hasten the deadly process of tissue destruction.

To get rid of an abscess, eat natural foods, especially those rich in citric acid, as lemons, oranges, grapefruit; strawberries and cherries are good, too. The black variety of cherry is especially valuable for hard tissue diseases like gall stones, gravel, cataract of the eyes, while red cherries are often used to break up general membranous conditions. Take fruits in the morning and at noon, and roots at night. Fruits are better eliminators than vegetables, which are primarily builders. Wastes have to be eliminated before the body can be built up; so start out the first week on the two meals of fruit and one of vegetables each day. You may eat nuts if you care to so as not to get hungry before the next meal. Eat real nuts along with your morning and noon meals, and peanuts at night. If you eat nuts with fruit, you should flake them, but if you wait for two hours, that will not be necessary.

If you have an ulcer or abscess that you can get at, whether external or in the rectum or vaginal region, make a pad of lemon and apply it as best you can. That will help kill the pus. Lemons are an enemy to pus; they will neutralize it instantly. You may feel a burning pain for just a little while upon application, but the end will be good. Give yourself lemon rubs, sponging yourself daily for a time with a mixture of lemon juice and water. Lemon is not like salves, liniments, etc., which seem to heal the outside but really only hinder the pus from coming out. In addition, drink all the lemon juice you want; it will bring the waste matter out of the blood and will destroy all threatening conditions within. Take it in warm water, quite sour.

ACIDITY

Q. Is the lemon ever the cause of acidity?

A. Lemon is the strongest acid there is, and if you have acidosis, acid is needed to cure it. Remember that the acid of the natural raw food is not acid in your stomach, for it will change to alkalinity within a few seconds after you eat it. A lemon in your mouth will be sour and astringent, but in your stomach, where the air is shut away from it, the sour changes to sweet. If you merely keep the mouth closed on it, you will notice that the sour has changed over to sweet. No natural raw fruit or raw acid can cause acidosis, but cooked acid is very dangerous. Cooked tomatoes and cooked rhubarb are a good source of acidosis. Do not be afraid of natural acids. They are all wholesome, good, clean, and strengthening, but cooked acids will not change except to sour, ferment, and finally turn into alcohol. They must be worked over so long by the stomach that some of the mixture is even changed into ether.

Q. How can acid stomach be most quickly over-come?

A. People want to do things quickly. We all do, but you will have to grow out of the trouble just as you grew into it. It took years to get acidosis; it may be years before the natural alkaline-acid balance in your body can be fully restored. Mix live food with patience and you will win every time.

Q. By what mistake in the raw food diet could one get too much acid in the system?

A. By taking acid fruits with cereals, starchy foods, and vegetables. If you mix fruit juices with cereals or starch, though these are raw, they will sour quickly and ferment. Never mix fruits with cereals, nor fruits with vegetables. Any acid vegetable or fruit when raw and eaten by itself will never cause acidosis.

Q. What is your remedy for hyperacidity?

A. Stop eating cooked acids. The difference between cooked and raw acids is this: the raw acid changes a few seconds after you swallow it, while the cooked acid is fixed and is not changed for hours afterwards. Only by evaporation can it be changed. The stomach cannot do this, so away goes the acid into the intestines, and then into the blood. That means acidosis. The stomach tries to alkalinize all foods before passing them on to the pyloris, a valve through which food escapes to the duodenum, thence to the small intestine. In a healthy digestive process, the stomach takes care not to allow acid to leave until changed to an alkali.

The food in the stomach must change to albumen in order to digest; therefore acid must become alkaline in the stomach to be prepared for assimilation.

Q. Is it true that acid blood condition can be cured in six months' time?

A. In passing, I will say that acidosis is not really too much acid, but rather too little alkalinity. I myself suffered from under alkalinity when I first tried this natural food. I lived on it 100 per cent for nine months before my blood gave the proper reaction. Many people will obtain a normal condition in six months. To find out where you stand, you don't need a doctor. Use litmus paper, obtainable at any drug store. Test it for yourself. Or try handling some poison oak. If your blood is really alkaline, there will be no bad effects.

Q. Are bicarbonate of soda and milk of magnesia of benefit to one suffering from acid stomach?

A. These two substances are drugs. As is the case with all drugs prescribed for human ailments by medical doctors, a beneficial reaction is often noted at the outset. With their continued use, however, the original trouble will become aggravated due to the necessity for the body's throwing out these very drugs, unassimilable and poisonous by their very nature. Specific cases are known where the sensitive lining of the stomach has actually been eaten away by these irritants. Depend for your stomach alkalinization upon Nature's simple, wholesome remedies—lemon juice, for example, and tomato juice.

ADENOIDS

Q. How can enlarged adenoids be cured?

A. Adenoids, also called pharyngeal tonsils, are found in children. The pharynx is the cavity back of the uvula, which in turn is above the throat. It is called the nasal cavity because the nose opens into it. In general, it is an opening or roomy space back of and above the mouth. The adenoids are a kind of gland which sometimes become oversized like tonsils and then close up the nasal cavity. That causes hard breathing, and operation is then usually resorted to for relief.

But adenoids can be reduced just as enlarged tonsils are reduced. You will generally find that children afflicted with adenoids like apples. If they do, just let them eat two or three apples immediately before bed time. Apples have a wonderful flavor, an enticing tartness, while the fumes attack the disease in the adenoids and tonsils, and cure them. Be sure you give the child no milk, no cheese, no eggs, meats, tea, coffee, or chocolate, but plenty of fruit juice in the morning. Let it have all the apples it wants, morning and night, and serve one meal of nice herbal salad together with some flaked peanuts. Peanuts go well with herbal salads; almonds blend well with fruits. Apples will cure the worst possible case of tonsilitis or adenoids. The swelling will soon go down and there will be no more trouble.

Should it be a long-standing case, one that is chronic, give the child hot and cold applications around the neck and throat. Put applications on for about fifteen or twenty minutes, hot and cold alternately, long enough so that plenty of blood can gather around the neck. Then teach the child to do these neck movements, each seven times:

1. Nod the head, as if to imply "yes."
2. Move the head from side to side, having in mind the ding-donging of a bell, the head being used for the striker.
3. Put chin over one shoulder, drop head over backwards, and so over to the other shoulder.
4. Give the head a sudden shake from right to left, quick turn.
5. Drop head down, turn it to the left, and, using the eyes to describe a circle, swing head around in circle seven times.
6. Drop head down and turn it to the right. Then swing it around in a circle, as above.
7. Drop head, bring 'way back, and shake it seven times.

In these exercises, the count should include an "and" between each figure as, 1 and, 2 and, 3 and, etc.

These exercises will help the blood to penetrate the affected muscular tissues. See that the child does them and is given the cold and hot applications every night before it goes to bed. This is a genuine cure. Natural foods, with the exercises, will cure any case of adenoids or tonsilitis.

Q. What is the cause and cure of adenoids?

A. The cause of tonsilitis and adenoids is wrong eating—too many carbohydrates, the cooked starches, and the flesh foods. There has been much wailing among marketeers and butchers: "Eat more meat; eat liver." What is it doing? Filling a multitude of graves. It is indigestible and merely putrifies in the stomach. What kind of blood can you expect to get in that way?

Q. My daughter, aged five, has very large adenoids, and I have been advised to have them removed. Is the operation necessary?

A. No. It is of little use to try to cure lameness by having the leg amputated. The adenoids are merely a swelling of the adenoid tissues in the nostrils, and, just as wrong living caused the swelling, right living will reduce the tissue to normal.

Q. I have heard you state that adenoids are largely the result of eating refined cereals and white bread. What, then, would you give a child for breakfast?

A. The breakfast food fad still has a tremendous hold on most people. They feel they could not live were they to have a breakfast without oatmeal or some other form of mangled grain. That is nonsense. A child will always have a favorite fruit, or fruits, which should be on the breakfast table every morning. The child should be allowed to help itself freely to whatever it desires, be it grapes, apples or peaches. Flaked nuts may be added in a side dish if desired. The adenoids of a child fed in this manner will become, or remain, normal.

ADHESIONS

Q. Can I remove adhesions by anything but operation?

A. If you have an adhesion, you must have had an operation prior to that. To overcome the adhesion, get some olive oil and lubricate the abdominal cavity just over where the adhesion hurts. Then put your finger tips there and pull on that adhesion. Stretch it as much as you can. Lie on your back with the knees up so that the abdominal cavity is flexible and soft. Work on the adhesion: stretch it right and left, and up and down, and rotate so that it will become longer. All this may hurt severely at times. Never mind, you are doing yourself good. You will stretch it so that soon it will not hurt at all. Do this at least once a day. You will not know, after a short time, that you ever had an adhesion.

Adhesions result from using the knife on some part of the body, and that itself is a good reason why you should never have operations performed. Adhesions make you suffer constant torture, a relentless tugging and pulling away. Do not have an operation, because another operation merely means another adhesion. Massage can, however, take it away in time. It will stretch the tissue sufficiently so that it will not trouble you. The sooner you start massaging after the operation, the better, for then the tissues are not so strongly knitted, and a little manipulation may even prevent trouble entirely.

ALCOHOL

Q. How can we cure a craving for alcohol?

A. Cooked sugar will supplant the craving of your body for liquor because it makes a still out of your stomach, where a genuine intoxicant is produced. The liquor habit is a false craving, just as much of a disease, in fact, as rheumatism or asthma, and the way to cure this craving is simply to live on natural food. I challenge anyone to live on natural foods for one year and then take a glass of whiskey without vomiting. I have treated the worst kind of drunkard and cured his passion for drink by simply putting him on a diet of raw fruits and vegetables.

Flesh foods are intoxicating on account of the ferments they cause. Ferments make men brutish, ferments of flesh foods especially, because this means uric acid in addition. Like associates with like—therefore you get so that you begin to crave liquor and tobacco, and begin to enjoy them. You need not try to convince your husband that the drinking of liquor is injurious—don't try it. Give him natural foods—take away the flesh foods and cooked meals, substituting raw fruits and vegetables, and then see how quickly you will have a nice, good-as-new husband. He will not smoke after nine months to a year of eating in this manner, and sometimes the reformation comes within a very few months. Neither men nor women can drink, or smoke, for that matter, if they live on natural foods. Why not live on preventive foods and be a strong, healthy, 100 per cent human being, instead of suffering from various diseases and false cravings, as well as being only about 15 or 20 per cent efficient?

Q. What is your stand on intoxicating liquor and tobacco?

A. Nowadays many men, and women as well, think they have to have a hot toddy or swallow whiskey, cocktails, or beer for an eye-opener. If they were raw food eaters, they could never take them. Any raw fooder who tries to drink liquor will find that it will come up as fast as he can put it down. The digestive organs have such strength and power that when anything as injurious as whiskey or any other alcoholic drink goes down, it will never in the world stay there. The stomach immediately refuses it. Just so will a clean body refuse tobacco, whether in the form of smoke or otherwise. Raw food would be, if generally recognized for its merits, an invaluable ally of all organizations fighting the liquor and tobacco habits.

Q. Will wine build the blood?

A. Only unfermented raw grape juice, or other pure fruit and vegetable juices, will give you the cell life for pure blood. The darkest grapes are the richest in iron. All wines are fermented; that is, alcoholic. If you must have something to drink with your meals, why not have a small glass of tomato, carrot, celery, orange, grapefruit, pomegranate, grape, or fresh apple juice? Coconut milk, too, is also very delicious. Choose the one which combines best with your meal.

Q. Do you approve of nursing mothers drinking beer to increase their milk flow?

A. Alcohol is a poison. It is true that the body manufactures for its own use a certain amount of natural alcohol required in the processes of metabolism. When the proper food is supplied, Nature will take care of this matter without any further aid. In the same manner, salt is supplied to the bloodstream by these processes of the body, without the necessity for eating any inorganic salt whatever. Nature is her own manufacturing chemist, supplying precisely the proportion required, and no more. Nursing mothers should, under no circumstances, indulge in alcoholic beverages. The sensitive internal tissues of the child are usually injured by even slight doses of poisonous substances taken either directly or indirectly. The mother herself requires to be in the best physical condition, and indulgence in alcohol will tear down and not build up. Animals, in an even tolerably natural environment, will always have a copious supply of milk.

ALUMINUM

Q. Some say aluminum ware is poisonous. Is that true?

A. Aluminum is not the best ware to use, but you would have to grind it up, or mill it, in order to get enough to be seriously poisoned. You would never get poisoned by merely eating from an aluminum spoon, or by boiling potatoes in an aluminum pot. That would not harm man enough to cause illness. All the same, it may cause trouble if constantly employed, just as when eating boiled potatoes and bread and butter daily. It is the continuous use that will finally harm you. Anyone who eats even an injurious substance today, but lets it go tomorrow, will not be hurt. If a person lives on natural foods he will soon be cleaned out again, but if he goes back permanently to eating cooked food, watch out! A live-fooder needs no pots and pans, and this matter is not a problem in his case, but cooked-fooders would do better to use agate ware, earthen, or iron ware.

Q. I have an aluminum roof plate in my mouth. Can this be damaging my body?

A. If you can be sure that the substitute is less, rather than more, poisonous, get rid of it. However, in these days of patent formulas, it is hard for the layman to be sure of anything as personal and important as a dental plate. The dentist who has knowledge of the natural way of living may be trusted, provided you can find him. I would be inclined to say that you should make a change, particularly if you have reason to suspect that something is wrong, something not traceable to any other cause.

ANÆMIA

Q. How do you cure pernicious anaemia?

A. Pernicious anaemia is a disease generally considered incurable. While all kinds of medical and non-medical doctors have been experimenting in methods of curing this disease, they have not been successful. Why not? Because the remedies they used are dead. These doctors allow their patients to partake of the cooked food they habitually eat. Furthermore, they fill them with drugs, also dead. Dead medicine and dead food are only disease builders. Drugs inhibit disease and some will take away pain, but they are not curatives.

The only remedies that will cure you are the ones that get the poisons and dead matter out of your body. When the body is clean, you are not only well, but are immune from any disease. Pernicious anaemia is dreaded as much as cancer, for it generally ends a person's life very quickly. Well, as long as there is life, there is hope. Let us never say die. Let us fight for life. No disease has any real power over our bodies if we put on our fighting clothes. Commence at once to live right in order to stop this disease from destroying any more of those red corpuscles. The blood contains two kinds of corpuscles—red and white. The white corpuscle belongs to an army of activity cells. The red corpuscle is the neutral part of the blood and must be replenished with the right kind of food. But when, in pernicious anaemia, you find that no blood is being made from the wholesome foods that you are eating, that the liver, spleen, and thyroid glands are not co-ordinating, that the food passes on without making blood, and the sunshine has no chance to cooperate, what are you going to do?

In such a case we must create red blood cells by induction; that is, the patient must be given the blood of an animal. Unnatural? True, but it is to save human life. Why not human blood? Friends, you cannot find a human being that has as good blood as an animal has. I would rather take chances with the animal. If I feed it, I will know that there will be blood material present that will induce the creation of red blood in the patient.

I had a patient once, a former blacksmith, who had pernicious anaemia. When I first came to his home he was in bed, being fed a little milk with oatmeal. I told the wife and daughter, who were his nurses, to get me about two dozen guinea pigs, to give them plenty of straw, and feed them on lettuce and spinach. After about three weeks, the animals were ready for the operation. In the meantime, we gave this man fruit juices, strawberries, beets, spinach, and carrots. We got our "piggies" ready. I obtained a tube eighteen feet long. I took two pigs up to the floor above, then ran the tube down, and put a nipple on it. I told the girl to take a cup, and, when she saw the blood come, to shut off the snapper, give the nipple to the father, and then to open it again. I went upstairs, shaved the neck of one of the "pigs," cut the jugular vein, and put a silver tube into it. The blood started flowing. It was not long before the guinea pig commenced to get weaker, so I took no more blood from it. The same procedure was repeated with another "pig," sending to the man more blood. We kept this up every day, and you ought to have seen how red he was. Every day we used new guinea pigs, until we had gone around the circle. By that time, the first were ready again. We kept it up until the man was restored to full health. He even commenced his blacksmithing again, and never required any more guinea pigs.

To explain what happened: the blood did not come in contact with the air at all. The patient got it directly from the "pig" into his stomach. His stomach passed it on to the body. This stimulated the thyroid gland and the spleen into creating blood of their own. I believe all foreign blood should go through the digestive tract so that it can be properly prepared by the various digestive fluids for transmission into the blood.

Q. What should I do for an anaemic condition? Everyone tells me I am very pale.

A. You need red blood; you have more white corpuscles than red—and you need sunshine, raspberry juice, beet juice, beet tops, and spinach—in short, all foods that contain the material to make good red blood. That includes all dark-colored reddish food, like beets, cherries, strawberries, prunes, plums, tomatoes. Of these, eat as much as you like, and with them a little honey and nuts. Try the real nuts with fruits, and peanuts with vegetables.

Q. Would you say there is a definite cause for anaemia?

A. Common anaemia is a term meaning a deficiency of blood, either in quality or quantity. There are two principal kinds of anaemia, first, common anaemia, where the blood lacks hemoglobin because of eating foods that destroy the red corpuscles. Certain cooked foods are especially destructive to red corpuscles, for instance the old-fashioned rhubarb pie. Rhubard pie, when baked, sets the acid in the rhubarb, cooked acid which destroys the red corpuscles. Another injurious food is stewed tomatoes. The tomato, in its natural state, is the finest of foods, but cooked, is one of the most dangerous, also because of this fixed acid. All kinds of acid fruit and vegetables that have been cooked are very bad for the blood. Strawberry pie, and jams and jellies made from acid fruits, are in this class. Meat eating, together with salt, help to cause anaemia. Salt is exceedingly destructive to the hemoglobin in the blood.

To overcome ordinary anaemia, simply stop eating cooked foods. That same tomato so dangerous when cooked, is very valuable when eaten raw. That cooked strawberry so destructive in a pie, is delicious and healthful in its natural state. So with the rhubarb. Extract the juice from rhubarb stalks, put in some honey, and you have the most delicious drink you can get, a drink that makes red blood.

Take sunbaths, too. Live in harmony with sunshine, for it is the sun, with right food, that gives you red blood. The sun, however, will make only waste matter out of dead food—it has no love for anyone who has dead food in him. Then it simply sours and destroys.

Q. My sister has anaemia. A New York specialist has advised her to eat red meats, such as liver. Will this enrich her blood?

A. Her blood will be "enriched" by the addition of nineteen grains of uric acid for every pound of liver eaten, and uric acid is a deadly poison. The body can rid itself, under normal conditions, of only three grains daily, and these are produced by the routine functioning of the organs. Any excess is eliminated only at the expense of extra wear and tear. Meat eating in itself is one of the chief causes of anaemia. There are so-called vitamines in liver, but why not get the same vitamines in fresh fruits and vegetables, without the necessity of absorbing at the same time the deadly uric acid?

APOPLEXY

Q. Will you tell us what causes apoplexy?

A. Apoplexy is sudden paralysis caused by an effusion or extravasation of blood in the brain, or by rupture in the spine. The effusion is caused by the rupture of a hardened vein or artery. This hardening of the blood vessel, in turn, comes from eating salt. Many different kinds of salt are taken in injurious quantities, not merely the usual sodium chloride or table salt, but, for example, alum, in cheap white bread, and bicarbonate of soda (baking powder) and cream of tartar in hot biscuits. Many people take baking soda to relieve gas in the system, or to cleanse the breath, which is a great mistake. Any salt substance that gets into the blood will bring hardening of the arteries, then paralysis, and sudden death.

Q. What is the best way to treat one suffering from apoplexy?

A. Probable over-excitement has strained an artery, the blood breaks through and deluges the lobe to the brain cells, and the man falls unconscious to the ground. Sometimes death comes instantly; sometimes the sufferer lives for three or four days. Again, he may survive, to have another attack later on if nothing is attempted in the way of remedy.

As first aid, soak a cloth in cold water and put it on his head. Call a doctor. The patient may have another hemorrhage within five days or on the fifth day. If he does, it is all up with him. The second one is generally fatal. As an aid to Nature, however, natural raw foods should be given the sufferer from the very beginning. Epsom salt baths are also helpful to draw the uric acid out of the system. Give gentle warm oil rubs and baths so as to cause skin absorption and take away the brittleness of the tissues. Feed him on nuts and dried olives as much as you can, since olives contain potassium and will help make tissue elastic. Be sure the olives are not salted or pickled in brine. These are absolutely dangerous. Only sun-dried black olives should be used. These are always dry when purchased and are sold in bulk only—never in cans or jars. It is salt that causes hardening of the arteries; therefore, salted olives would intensify the condition. During the period of illness, or while convalescing, the head should be kept quite cool, but alternate now and then with a warm (not hot) cloth. Long-continued illness will cause slowing down of the circulation, so always use warm applications in one warm to three cold alternation to give relief to the fixed vibration. For permanent cure, abstain from all salt eating; live on natural organic fruits, herbs, and roots. These contain no destructive mineral salts—all is organic and therefore beneficial.

APPENDICITIS

Q. Are appendix operations necessary?

A. Appendicitis is an inflammation of the vermiform appendix. A certain doctor once told me that the appendix is something like a rattlesnake: if it becomes inflamed you must get it out or it will kill you. What a terrible remark to make, to frighten people into operations. The appendix vermiform is really very useful. It is a little tail-like appendage at the bottom of the colon, next to where the ileum valve connects the small intestine with the colon. The appendix is lined with fatty glands that furnish the oil for the lubrication of the valve. The appendix may get inflamed, I admit, but many times when the case is diagnosed as appendicitis, it is really colitis. The colon is very likely to be inflamed—sometimes both are.

Appendicitis is brought on, usually, by eating cooked foods until the peristaltic action of the bowels has weakened to such an extent that you cannot have a normal bowel movement, or, in other words, you have constipation. Then congestion is felt when food is forced up into the ascending colon to the hepatic plexus. There the colon turns at a right angle toward the splenic plexus, then down, forming the sigmoid flexure, and finally the rectum. The large colon is about five feet long and full of globular villi. If you had lived on natural foods all your life, you would not now have constipation or appendicitis. You are suffering because you have failed to keep in line with Nature's law. Is it any wonder you get sick? It is really a wonder that people live as long as they do. The reason they get along at all is because of intestinal ferments which form gas enough to push the waste matter out of the bowels. You may think you are in good condition if you have one movement a day, but you are not. The villi are clogged and buried in their own waste matter, and the gas ferment of decayed food is necessary to push it through—in other words, mechanical bowel movement instead of peristaltic action.

Of course, Nature weakens continuously—you keep on getting worse. Finally, some of this colonic waste material breaks off and drops down in little hard clots toward the appendix. New matter coming up from the intestines through the ileum tries to work it up, but in vain. This mass of putrefaction crowds the valve which is keeping the door shut to anything returning to the small intestine. At last some works its way into the weakened appendix, causing it to distend. Soon there will be real inflammation there. Finally, it is so full it really hurts. Then we are told it has to be cut out. I know better. I had in Minneapolis, in 1913 and 1914, over 300 cases diagnosed as appendicitis by doctors. These all came to me because they heard that I cured without operating, and all were cured by my drugless, knifeless method. None had adhesions later because I did not operate on them.

Q. How can chronic appendicitis be cured?

A. A masseur, or any man who is clever with his hands, can do much to aid Nature in curing appendicitis. The first thing to do, however, is to clean out the bowel thoroughly with enemas. Then give the bowel a good lubrication with oil. After you have filled it with oil and the oil has been discharged, put the patient on his back, raise the hips as high as you can, and let the feet hang back over so that they will not draw the muscles. Then the masseur should lubricate his hands and commence by rotating them over the appendix. With the fingers of one hand, press upward to the hepatic plexus. The fingers will slip very easily because the skin has been well oiled. Press right over the colon and keep vibrating as you slip your fingers up, so as to induce a vacuum. The head being lower causes everything to come up out of the appendix by mere action of gravity. Now alternate hands and keep up this massage until you are sure you have caused a vacuum in the colon, which, when there, will suck

everything out of the appendix. The oil which you
have placed inside will cause a good sealing, or cohe-
sion of the walls of the colon, so that no air will come
back. In this way, try to get the substance into the
transverse colon. It will be only a little, as the appendix is small—only about the size of the little finger.
You cannot get very much in it, but only a trifle there
may hurt a great deal. You may require much massaging in order to get that trifle out, but it will be worth
while, and you may rest assured it will not get in again
if the patient will consistently live on raw food.

APPETITE

Q. Should one who gets up late and has no appetite
for three meals daily, eat only two meals, and what
should they consist of?

A. If a person has no appetite and wants to eat only
one meal per day, it is all right, even though our civli-
ization has adopted the customary three, irrespective
of whether hungry or not. The right way is to eat when
you are hungry. When you are not hungry, do not eat.
When you eat, eat until your hunger is stilled, and
then stop. Do not measure the quantity of food—let
your tastebuds measure it. When you want to eat, select
that which seems most delicious to you, for that will
digest most perfectly and will do you the most good.

Q. I have been living on raw food for several weeks
but I am very hungry. How long will this last?

A. If you are very hungry, eat. Some people have
starved themselves so long on cooked material that

when they commence to eat real food they seem famished. When you get your body reconstructed, you will not be constantly hungry. In fact, you will eat so little that people will wonder how you can do so much work on such modest rations. It will be because you are eating 100 per cent live foods.

ARTHRITIS

Q. How can one cure arthritis?

A. First we must get at the cause. For all the twenty-seven different kinds of arthritis, there is but a single great cause; namely, salt eating. It makes no difference where or how you get this salt into your system, whether in large quantities or small; in time your body will become saturated with it. Dead foods of course will not go down without the addition of salt. Your tastebuds rebel. They are calling for real food—uncooked fruits and vegetables. Gratify them. See that you get plenty of exercise. Bathe daily. Stimulate your muscles to throw off the impurities collected there. The more you perspire by exercise in the sunshine, the quicker you will get rid of your arthritis. Also put on a poultice of potatoes and onions where afflicted, alternating with flaxseed.

Q. What can be done for arthritis deformans?

A. When you see your joints getting large, it is high time to ask that question. You must first dissolve the salt in your joints. Make a pair of little bags into which you can put your hands, or your feet, or get some thick stockings or socks. Prepare a poultice of onions and raw potatoes ground fine. Grind them with a vegetable grinder, then mix them, and put enough into your bag or stocking so that there will still be room for your hands or feet. Tie it well above the ankle or wrist. Have a string through it like a sack, and draw it tight at the top. Then for something to keep the juice from coming through. Use a paper bag for that. A twenty pound sugar bag will be all right. That will finish the job. Go off to bed and leave the wrapping on all night. Next morning take it off and wash the leg or arm thoroughly. Also wash out the bag and hang it on the line to dry. The next night do the same thing. Keep that up regularly.

Remember that arthritis is a very difficult disease to cure because you have to dissolve a deposit in your joints. When this is dissolving, you are going to have pains, as in rheumatism. Why? Because of the uric acid which was first eaten in food. This gave you rheumatic pains. These were caused by acid then in your blood. Later, the acid settled in the joints. This uric acid, by and by, changed into urates, really salt by reason of age. The uric liquid has evaporated and left only the sediment of salt in the joints. Now, when you commence to live on natural food and vegetable juices, the urates dissolve and are redeposited in the blood. You will perhaps blame the juices for giving you rheumatism, but oranges never gave anyone rheumatism. They only reliquify deposited urates in order to get them out of the system.

You must get the waste matter out. When you are starting a furnace fire, you must first clean out the ashes, put in kindling and fuel, and then you will have a nice clean fire. So with the fire of life in your body. You must clean out of the furnace all debris that has been deposited there by unnatural foods. Neither fever nor perspiration will take it out—nothing but living as Nature intended you should. You must live on live foods and use natural juices as beverages between meals. You must give your body the organic salt it needs.

After two or three weeks of poulticing, change from onion-potato to flaxseed. Get some ground flax meal, put some into your bags, and dip into boiling hot water. Then take them out and let cool long enough so that you can comfortably put your hand into them. Tie just as you did the other poultice. Do that for two or three nights and then commence using half onion and potato, half flaxseed meal. The flaxseed poultice will furnish the lubricant and will take away the extreme skin dryness. Patience and endurance will be very essential, but you will be rewarded by complete freedom from arthritis.

This reconstruction work may cause an affliction of the heart for the period of the elimination, because all blood that is saturated with uric acid and other wastes will also affect the heart. Do not be alarmed. The fresh juices and other raw foods will counteract this condition. Drink as much natural fruit juice as you care to. Choose quantity, as well as variety, by taste.

Q. What foods are best to eradicate a gouty condition?

A. All natural foods that contain natural salts are

good to eradicate arthritis deformans, or gouty rheumatism.

Q. What is the best way to get rid of bad joint rheumatism?

A. To cure rheumatoid arthritis, put hot applications on the joints so as to get your blood there—the best possible healer. The next thing is, seeing to it that the blood gets the proper reconstruction material, and that comes only from natural food. Nothing else can make better blood to give and maintain perfect health. Never rub a swollen joint because you will make it worse. Give your body an Epsom salt bath twice a week. Poultice the joints with onions and potatoes, and now and then with flaxseed meal. Exercise every day.

ASTHMA

Q. What is the best treatment for asthmatic conditions in a seventy-year-old woman, and what is the cause?

A. Asthma is a catarrhal condition which is generally brought on by the eating of flesh foods and dairy products, especially flesh. That is where you get your catarrh, which is a very disagreeable thing at the best. Asthma makes you hunger and strain for air, but the phlegm coating your nostrils, bronchial tubes, and all your lung cells, shuts off most of it. That is asthma. Remember, you cannot live long without air.

You want to know what to do in case you get one of those attacks? First, bring your head down to your chest. Then bring your head backward as far as you can. Open the mouth and inhale. Finally exhale with the mouth open. Anyone with an attack of asthma coming on can break it up instantly by this method, for when you raise your head far back the muscles which are fastened to the mastoid bones and to the clavicle, lift the ribs. That allows the lungs more room to expand, and when you breathe you can stretch every lung cell. You will no longer choke for want of air, since some of the cells will respond to the exercise, and you will be relieved. It is true that you will commence to cough, but that is precisely what we want. It will bring that phlegm out. Next, clasp your hands, bringing the elbows up to the side, and pound the side with the elbows, expelling short breaths of air at the same time. That little jarring in the lung cells causes the phlegm to break loose. More coughing will result, and more expelled phlegm. If the lungs feel sore afterwards it is well to try to get some mint, such as spearmint, and inhale it. Practice these exercises every day, and in addition, do not forget—no more dead carcass in the stomach, no more milk, cheese, butter, or eggs, the cause of all phlegm diseases.

Epsom salt baths are valuable. Put two pounds of Epsom salt into a bathtubful of blood-warm water. Soak in it for ten minutes, after which rub with a cold sponge or towel all over to get off the coating on the skin. Then soak another ten minutes in the water and rub again. Repeat this a third time. Drain the tub and get under a cold shower, or, if there is none, take a bath towel and rub with cold water for about a minute, so as to close the pores of the skin and prevent catching cold. The baths will stimulate and help to do away with the asthmatic condition. Keep this up every day until the phlegm is out of the system.

Sunbaths are also very good. Exercise while you sunbathe, and take a warm bath lasting fifteen minutes to one-half hour immediately afterward. Finish with a cold rub-down. Do this between the hours of nine and twelve A.M., and increase the time spent in the bath from a half hour to one hour. In this manner the worst form of asthma can be cured.

Q. A lady is suffering from asthma and is very weak. The coughing is driving her to despair. Can anything be done to cure her?

A. The coughing is a very good sign. When a person has power enough to cough, even though he does not get up anything at the time, it is a splendid indication that he has strength enough to throw off the impurities. Tickling will induce coughing. This will be accomplished by putting into the mouth a teaspoonful of honey. Do not swallow it, but let it draw the saliva to the mouth from the salivary glands. There may be a sore spot in the throat or in the tonsils which irritates and produces this coughing. Let the mouth fill with saliva; then spit it all out. Take some distilled water, gargle, and then wash out the mouth. Take another teaspoonful of honey and do exactly the same thing, and continue doing this until it seems very difficult to get any more saliva. About three or four times will do the work very nicely. Then take a drink of some good fruit juice. Epsom salt baths, too, will help in this case.

Q. What food should you give for asthma?

A. Eat natural foods and you will get well again. Eat those fruits in the morning which you like best, leafy vegetables at noon, and roots at night. Honey is one of the best agents for getting phlegm out of the system, so eat it freely in the case of asthma, hay fever, and other catarrhal diseases. Do not touch dairy products, tea, coffee, chocolate, alcohol, or tobacco.

Q. How long will it take to clear up a case of asthma?

A. It may take from nine months to two and a half years before you can get the catarrhal waste out of the system. Everything depends upon the severity of the disease and the thoroughness with which you set about to cure it. Although I have known patients to recover in nine months' time, one gentleman under my care had his first crisis of elimination after about two years. But keep at it 100 per cent and you will find your breathing power improving constantly.

AUTO-INTOXICATION

Q. Give the cause of severe auto-intoxication and what initial diet and progressive changes in diet are necessary to establish normal health; also the length of time required to do so.

A. Auto-intoxication affects every individual in a way peculiar to himself. Consequently, every individual must find his own remedy. Everyone will discover the natural food which tastes best to him, as well as the amount to eat and how often. After a month or two, you will have learned much about yourself and your needs; the value of live food measured by your improvement will be conspicuous. Careful experimentation, flavored with patience, is essential in any process of getting well, for it is going to take almost as long to get well as it took you to get sick. If you have many aches and pains or have been doing much smoking, drinking, etc., it is going to take you much longer to "snap out of it" than it will the person who has lived a more or less wholesome life. Nature knows in detail what has to be done. You can, if you do your part faithfully, leave the rest to her. There is no short-cut to health.

BACTERIA AND GERMS

Q. Are bacteria and germs dangerous to health?

A. Bacilli and germs are minute cells that cannot be seen unless they are magnified from 500 to 1000 diameters with a microscope. The rod-shaped tuberculosis bacilli go usually in pairs. Sometimes bacilli are connected like a chain, as in anthrax. All these germs or bacilli are our friends, inasmuch as they eat waste matter that has collected in our system. This process generally causes irritation, but why do we have so much waste matter in the first place? If we would eat live food, clean foods, waste matter would never pile up thus. Therefore we would not carry about any microbes, disease germs, or bacteria.

We need never be alarmed about these organisms as long as we live on natural foods, for fruits and nuts and vegetables never produce waste matter. Therefore they cannot furnish food for parasites. Sunshine, or even electric light, if it is strong enough, will destroy tuberculosis bacilli in from two to five seconds. This germ will often infest the normal lung cells. You may find it in a healthy lung since there may be a little waste matter or phlegm there in which it can live. When, however, you supply your body with natural live foods, phlegm will get out of you just as quickly as it can. The bacilli will not have time to dig into your organs before being thrown out. It is not so with people who live on cooked foods, for ,their membranous tissues are weakened, are very tender, have no dynamic force, no power, and therefore the tuberculosis bacilli will have food, a place for activity, and will set up considerable irritation, without causing a cough or being interrupted in their work. There is in these people a universal lack of dynamic energy, lack of internal cleanliness, lack of the "dyno" force of mucous membranous tissue all through the internal tissues of the digestive tract and lungs.

Q. Are germs the cause of infectious diseases such as typhoid or diphtheria?

A. No, they are the result, rather than the cause. They are the result of the heaping up of waste matter in the body, and aid in its summary removal. The crisis in such process of removal is then called an infectious disease. The term "infectious" implies that large numbers of people go through the same cleaning process at approximately the same time, due, it may be, to meteorological and general conditions as much as to any actual contact with the germs.

BATHING

Q. Some people advise only infrequent bathing. What do you think of this?

A. Any disease, I do not care which you mention, can be eliminated much more quickly with the aid of one, two, or three baths a day than without them. Diseases are caused by accumulated filth, and the more baths you take, the faster you get rid of this waste matter. Some people think they are very clean because they have a clean shirt, clean underwear, and everything externally is washed. Not necessarily so. You may have clean clothes, yes, but they cannot clean your skin. They really prevent the sun and wind from drying it out. It would then scale off as it is renewed from beneath. The only way, then, because we do wear clothes, is to take many more water baths. The wearing of clothes is really very poor policy. It hides the deformity and lack of development that we are unconsciously ashamed of.

When we wake up in the morning, one of the first things to do is to drink a glass of water. Then a good cold shower bath, or cold sponge bath, should be taken. This is not much of a cleanser—it is more of a tonic—but very good. It stimulates the blood circulation and nerve force. It also clears the brain. By giving yourself a good towel rub or self-massage afterward, you stimulate the circulation and help the heart. All this is the process of helping waste to be eliminated through the skin, and when you are eating natural food, its natural force within the stomach helps by working from within outward, for there is a dynamic energy in all living food.

Q. What kind of bath do you advise for the morning?

A. Take a lukewarm shower bath and finish up by turning on the hot water, then the cold, hot again, and finally cold. Do this every day. If you can stand all cold water without undue chilling, that is to be preferred.

Q. How do you take an Epsom salts bath?

A. Put two pounds of Epsom salt in a bathtubful of blood-warm water; that is, about 100 degrees Fahrenheit. After you have been in the bath ten minutes, you will feel a kind of slime on your skin. Step out, and with a sponge of cold water, rub off this slime. Then get back into the water for another ten minutes. Rub off the slime as before, and continue in this manner until there appears to be no more slime. Three times, perhaps, and you will have cleaned it off fairly well. Now change the water. Draw off the blood-warm water and fill the tub with cold. Meantime, prepare your towel, so that when you get through with the cold water you can take your rub and go to bed, for this should be the last bath of the day. When the tub is full of cold water, put one foot in slowly, then the other, and gradually slip in. You will not like it very well at first, but you will get used to it. Go right down under. Then get out, rub yourself with the towel, and go to bed.

Blood-temperature water with Epsom salt in it will

open the pores of the skin and coax the poisonous uric acid out. Always take a cold sponge after each ten-minute period of the Epsom salt bath, finishing the third period with a cold dip. In fact, any bath should employ cold water as the finishing touch. Epsom salt baths are good for rheumatism. Always keep the water at blood heat, or the pores will close. Besides, for permanent relief, take natural protein—lettuce, spinach, cauliflower, beets, and the fruits all contain it.

Q. Is it all right to take Russian sweat baths?

A. Do not take Russian sweat baths or Turkish baths; they merely weaken you. Only strong people can really endure them. Take an Epsom salts bath instead. Sweat baths are very good when you produce them by working your muscles in the sunshine, but if you do not, as in the Russian bath, you are eliminating the best element of the blood while the worst remains in the body. Remember that all kinds of sweat baths must be accompanied by exercises or else you will lose quantities of the best fluid in the system. With Epsom salts baths you may lie as still as you care to, because the impurities are brought out by chemical affinity.

Q. Is a sulphur bath in a hot, natural spring healthy?

A. No, the fumes of sulphur are not good for you.

Q. What is your opinion on the various types of baths?

A. "Hydro" means water; "therapy," its therapeutic or curative value. When you merely hear someone say "water cure," very little impression is made upon your mind. You do not see how water can cure anything. You bathe yourself daily, wash your face and hands, you drink water, and that is all you know about it. You think that its curative value is nil because you use it daily in a simple way. You have probably never thought of heating the water and causing a hyperemia, and you have probably never thought of taking a continuous bath lasting from one to three hours. You have not thought of taking baths at short intervals, or for different conditions; for your head, your heart, or perhaps the whole body, with possibly the aid of salt, or sodium; Epsom salt, or magnesium sulphite. You do not hear me say "sulphur." That is not a desirable element in which to bathe. We often depend upon water alone in its different temperatures. Remember, it is not so much the water as its therapeutic value through thermic changes through heat and cold. These make a splendid force of stimulus and reaction. The hot water will bring the blood to the surface; the cold water will cause it to retreat again.

It also closes the pores of the skin, and thus is more of a tonic. One of the best and quickest tonics is called the Scotch douche. The operator puts you into a little square all closed in with marble slabs and braced up so that the water cannot get through. He has two helpers; one has a blanket and the other a sheet. They stand on each side of the opening, and the operator about ten or twelve feet back. He takes a hose and turns on the lukewarm water. He knows just how to manipulate it, while the helpers will watch the individual and tell him to turn about just as the operator directs. First they commence on the face. The operator knows how to manage the hose, which has sixty pounds pressure to every square inch. The water is dashed up against the body, but he is careful not to strike the stomach, the lower abdomen, and certain parts of the face. It is essential to avoid striking the cervical of the neck, even for a moment. The heat of the water meantime is gradually increased. After the patient has turned about face three or four times, the water has become hot. A thermometer informs the operator of the exact temperature of the water. After about 110 degrees is registered, the operator suddenly turns on ice water. You can imagine the patient's shock. He will be quickly turned about so as to get the water on the back and front at the same time. Then one of the attendants with a sheet, and the other with a blanket, will lay him on the massage table and begin to massage. You may come for your douche in just as tired, and sore, and worried a state as you please. Go through that bath and you will forget all about your condition. You will be able to walk ten miles or have a good tussle. You will feel as though you had never been tired at all. That is all done with water. The force of the spray will have made your skin a rosy pink.

Q. Is ocean-bathing beneficial, or is it harmful because of the salt? Do you favor swimming as an exercise?

A. Ocean water contains the same elements as the human blood, minus only the red corpuscles—so say some authorities. The craving for a dip in the ocean may thus go back to past milleniums in the history of the human race, may satisfy a deep and primeval craving. Apart from this, however, the stimulating effect of the cold water dashing against the body, is a desirable one. The salt itself need not be feared, since too little of it is absorbed through the pores to make any appreciable difference. The fresh air that sweeps in over the ocean is also an active agent in health building.

Swimming is considered by some physical trainers to be the most ideal form of exercise, involving all the muscles and organs. Indoor pools, however, are to be shunned, not only as the air is generally foul, but also because of the chlorine with which the health boards require the water to be doped. This does not mean that everyone, indiscriminately, should be forced to learn to swim, for some have an instinctive repugnance to water. These individuals should first build up their general vitality, and then there will be time enough for sports. Nature is often wiser than we think, and her instincts should be respected.

BLADDER

Q. What causes weakness of the bladder or a frequent desire for urination? How can I obtain relief?

A. The cause of this weakness is eating food with plenty of salt and vinegar, as well as sugar and candy. That weakens the tissues all the way down to the bladder. There are three remedies, all common and very good. Try watercress. It grows in any mountain stream

(from which you may gather it yourself), or it may
be purchased at large fruit and vegetable markets. If
you find that when you take watercress alone your
bladder burns at night, hurts you so much that you
cannot tell whether or not you are urinating, then mix
some lettuce with it. Use half lettuce and half watercress. If that has alleviated the burning sensation so
that you can take your herbs without nagging and
burning, you have the proper procedure. But I would
advise you to wear a napkin, especially at night. Keep
this up until there is no more burning sensation. Increase the cress and decrease the lettuce until you can
take the watercress alone without the familiar symptom of burning. When you can do that, you are almost
well. You will find that by eradicating the catarrhal
condition with the cress, your bladder will be well
under control. The same results may be accomplished
if nasturtium leaves or mustard greens are used in
place of the watercress. Try all three herbs and see
which you like best. Sometimes, of course, we have to
take that which we can get. Both nasturtium and
mustard greens are easily grown, so perhaps you can
raise your own in your back yard or garden.

In addition to the above, a hot sitz-bath should be
taken every night before retiring, one of progressive
heat, which means sitting in it as warm as you can bear,
adding hot water to the point of endurance. When you
have been in the bath for about twenty-five minutes,
turn on the cold water for one minute. Then rub down
and go to bed. This is the technique for the cure of
weakness in the bladder of babies, children, and grown-
ups; catarrh of the bladder; enlarged prostate, and

all forms of urethral trouble. It also helps in venereal diseases.

Q. Will you please tell me what to do for bed wetting. I wake up at night and my bed is wet. I have no dreams and no warning. I have had this since I was a child.

A. You have a catarrhal bladder. This organ has become insensitive. The catarrh has coated its exit to the extent that the sensory nerves cannot indicate a desire or lack of desire for urination. Therefore the bladder has lost its power to retain the urine. Eat some lettuce and watercress, half and half, once a day; at noon is the best time. Take some olives immediately after every meal, as many as you enjoy. If you do not like them, take only as many as you can without their nauseating you. Watercress will cause a burning sensation in the bladder. This salad, then, every day until you can eat straight watercress without discomfort. That means you are cured. You will have discharges, in the course of the treatment, of catarrhal mucous from the bladder, but consider this a normal part of your progress. Finally the catarrhal condition will be removed and the sphincter muscles at the neck of the bladder closed just like a lock, and they will not open until you want them to. Should the lack of control ever recur, you will soon get relief by taking a little watercress. You may have to do that until you have lived 100 per cent on live food long enough to have strengthened the muscles and eliminated the catarrhal condition permanently.

Q. My urine contains a stringy, cloudy matter. What can be done? Will fasting help?

A. No, not yet. That is an indication of an inflammation that contains pus. You must have sharp or stinging pains in your urethra or bladder, like the cutting of a knife or the prick of a pin or needle. Your drinks, whatever they are, should be rich in lemon juice and honey. Lemon juice will destroy the pus germ and the honey will draw it out of the system. Use plenty of greens or other vegetables.

Q. What should be the color of healthy urine?

A. Urine should be a light straw color.

Q. When I eat much fruit, the urine irritates and causes me considerable pain in the bladder.

A. If you like these fruits you have been eating, but they irritate and cause pain in the bladder, then keep right on eating them, only in smaller quantity. If possible, dilute the food. Take with it a drink of water or something else that has not the same acidity. For instance, if you are eating an apple, mix with an avocado—and eat less, too. Mix well with saliva.

Q. What does blood in the urine indicate?

A. Blood in the urine indicates one of several things. It may be that you have simply an abrasion in the urethra or in the channel through which the blood passes, caused by wrong treatment for certain venereal diseases. It may also be that you have an inflammation, or even an ulcer, in the bladder, that is discharging and possibly bleeding. You may notice the blood but not the catarrhal element, although they are distinct in color. These organs may bleed and yet you would not feel any pain—only nausea because of the loss of blood. Another cause of internal bleeding is food that forms pus—all animal foods, especially those richly flavored with pepper and salt. There may also be a broken blood vessel in the kidneys or bladder.

We must do something to stop this bleeding. Inject a natural astringent into the penial organ and see if that will not heal it. This liquid may be expected to draw the tissues together. I can recommend one liquid especially, and that is, well-strained lemon juice. Use with equal parts of water warmed to about blood heat. Put into a fountain syringe and catheterize into the penial organ. Let it discharge as freely as it wants to. This will purify and strengthen the diseased condition. If it is an ulcer, it will certainly be cured. Do this twice a day.

Q. My urine is sometimes dark and heavy. Please tell cause and cure.

A. You have evidently a feverish condition somewhere in the urinal tract, either in the bladder or in the kidneys, but most likely in the bladder and the urethra. This fever affects the urine and gives it a dark red color. Drink plenty of water and raw juices. Lemon will help to allay the inflammation. Cucumbers and tomatoes, half and half, are the finest remedies for these troubles. Watermelon is also very helpful.

Q. What will relieve bladder irritation?
A. It is relieved very quickly by warm-water flush-

ing of the bladder. It is well to put a little glycerine into the water, probably a teaspoonful to a cup of water. Stir thoroughly; have it about blood warm. Get a small catheter that goes in easily, and slowly put so much water into your bladder that it will wash back outside of the catheter. Flush once a day, and the irritation will disappear. Now to get at the cause of the irritation. You may have been eating watercress, mustard greens, or some other kind of stimulant, and it may have affected the neck of the bladder. If that is the case, keep right on. It proves you have a weakness there. A hot sitz-bath for half an hour is also good. Finish with a cold rub. These baths should be taken just before bed time.

Q. I have continual pain in the bladder; also urinate too often; have temperature. Explain, please.

A. Fill a bathtub with hot water. Have the water as hot as you can bear it, and when you feel yourself getting dizzy, put a cold cloth around your head and drink a swallow of cold water now and then. After twenty minutes or half an hour, get out and rub cold water all over the hips as high as the hot water has reached. Then lie on your back.

BLOOD

Q. What foods are best as blood builders?

A. You will find that strawberries, lettuce, spinach and the cresses, chicory, parsley, are all good blood builders; also dark fruits, such as prunes, etc., have good blood-building qualities.

Q. What causes a rather violent beating in the abdominal region, usually noticed when in bed in the morning?

A. This is aneurysm, a dilation which forms on the side of the artery, the great aorta. This large artery sometimes weakens in spots, due to too high temperature, and bulges out. Then the blood going through is impelled, and you will hear it pulsating like a hammer. The aorta goes around the neck like the handle of a cane, then divides and runs into the arms and legs. You can feel it where it approaches the stomach. The cure is to cleanse your body and to purify it. Take frequent baths and good, wholesome food. Put a bandage around your waist snug enough so that when you are standing up it will correct and steady the nerves and not allow such strong vibrations. Manipulate the aneurysm with your fingers to squeeze out the bulging. When this is done, the pulsation goes, too. Use a rotary hand motion. Lying on your back, press as deeply as you can with one finger, and rotate toward the right. When you get to where the beating is located, take your other hand and push the aneurysm out. The aorta soon becomes as elastic as rubber, while under the old method of living it gets brittle. The rotation will help the condition, but remember to wash and bathe to get the poison out. Sunshine is a wonderful help in such a case.

Q. Please tell me what function carbon fulfills in the body.

A. Excess carbon is waste matter, while carbon

dioxide or monoxide is used tissue salt. Your blood goes round and gathers this up. When it gets back to the lungs, the carbon dioxide and the bisulphate of sodium will be expelled through the nostrils.

Q. What foods will build red blood?

A. Lettuce is rich in iron; spinach in sodium and chloride; cabbage in calcium; and beet root is wonderful as a night food, as is the carrot. The turnip is better for the dentyne and enamel of the teeth, while the beet is best for blood building. Beet root also has protein, coloring matter. It will furnish color for your hair if you are gray. Do not wear a hat. The best blood is possible only when the sun shines on your entire body. Take as many clothes off as feasible and work in the garden. Work barefooted, and in shorts, without shirt or hat. Let the sun take hold of you, at first for about ten minutes; increase the next day to fifteen minutes, and keep on until you can stay out all day without discomfort. Sunshine and live food go well together.

BLOOD POISONING (GANGRENE)

Q. Tell me what to do for a sore on the heel when gangrene has set in.

A. Gangrene is flesh rot. This is not a light matter; we must give you prompt aid. Get some of the greenest looking herbs you can find—lettuce, the leafy kind which is most tender, not head lettuce. Mash it up into a pulp and put it on your heel in the form of a poultice twice a day. If the heel is not too sore, you might put into each poultice, after mixing it up thoroughly, about one teaspoonful of lemon juice. This will increase the antiseptic power. All the while, be careful to live on natural foods one hundred per cent and get your blood revitalized. Get plenty of sunbaths; also a lukewarm to hot to cold shower bath daily.

BLOOD PRESSURE—HIGH AND LOW

Q. How do you treat high blood pressure?

A. High blood pressure comes from eating high protein foods, like animal flesh and animal products such as milk and eggs. High blood pressure is dangerous in cases of hardening of the arteries, causing apoplexy. Begin by asking yourself, how did I get sick? There is a cause for every illness. Check your daily routine critically. Mornings you may be going through a daily dozen, taking warm and cold shower baths and a glass of orange juice. All very good. Then at breakfast you have a cup of coffee. That is all right, you think; everybody else drinks it—your great grandmother, your grandmother, your mother. Why not you? Yet one generation may have had rheumatism, the next generation rheumatism, Bright's disease and dropsy, and the next generation may die young. Yet we wonder why. It is because of this same routine of living on degenerated foods. Coffee contains the equivalent of three grains of uric acid in the form of caffeine and tannin. Then you add high proteins in milk; you stir in some sugar, which is harmful since it is made by the boiling process. There, in sum, you have the ordinary cup of coffee, a real disease builder. What good can that glass of orange juice do?—not a great deal, because the acids created by the coffee will have to be partially neutralized by the live orange juice. Everything that has been prepared by fire or processed in any way, is a disease builder. One who has lived on live food for a year and works or sleeps outside, will have a healthy complexion and plenty of red blood. You can distinguish the live-food eater from the cooked-fooder by his velvety skin texture. The skin of the cooked-fooder will be rough and pasty. The right way to keep free from high blood pressure is to live on normal foods. First of all, then, eliminate from your daily menu and routine those things which caused the blood pressure to be high.

Q. What is good for high blood pressure? I am a lady forty-seven, going through change of life.

A. High blood pressure is caused by a superabundance of filth in the blood. The more filth there is, the more ferment; the more ferment, the more gas, the more pressure. Blood pressure varies with the activity of the body. Let the doctor put his instrument on your arm and take the pressure. Suppose he finds it low. Then run around the block, come right back, and let him take the pressure again. It will be high. Just running around the block will do that. Besides this obvious objection, we do not know what the normal blood pressure really is—we have no normal standard to measure by, for we haven't anyone who is normal as yet. Live the best you know how—getting man's proper food, plenty of exercise, fresh air, sunshine, and rest, and your blood pressure will soon get back to what it should be.

Q. What diet is good for high blood pressure?

A. Sufferers from high blood pressure must keep away from milk, butter, cheese, eggs, and flesh foods. They should eat the natural greens and fruits, and among these those which contain the least amount of protein. The avocado is one of these, with only about two per cent protein. All nuts are fairly rich in protein, also all legumes. So keep away from the legumes and nuts for a while, but eat all the lettuce, spinach, celery, and other herbs that you want. Some of them, ture, are rich in chlorophyll protein, which, however, is harmful only if cooked. When uncooked, these herbs are the best food you can get. They will never cause high blood pressure, and will provide you with living salts. Spinach is the richest of all these in both sodium and chloride, in this form an absolutely non-crystalliz-ing salt.

Q. Am a strict raw-fooder. Blood pressure is below normal. Is there any danger? Am feeling well. What will bring the blood up to normal?

A. Raw food; nothing else. Do not be alarmed about low blood pressure, but be alarmed when it is too high. Quick movements will soon restore you to normal. Your body needs to be stirred up a bit, that's all.

BOILS AND CARBUNCLES

Q. What would you advise for one suffering from anthrax?

A. Anthrax is a malignant carbuncle; in other words, a cancer in the shape of a carbuncle usually appearing in the most sensitive part of the body—the back of the neck. Anthrax is the result of unclean blood, of waste matter accumulated in the neck tissues. It is often brought about by the wearing of furs around the neck. The dye gets into the pores of the skin when the furs become moistened with snow or rain. That also happens to the dye or coloring in feather boas when you are caught out. This dye, of course, produces irritation and finally forms a growth which finds food in the tissue waste matter beneath. In shape, the growth is like a common carbuncle, but very vicious and painful, generally leaving a great hole after losing its core. Anthrax is impossible when one goes bare-necked and lives on natural foods.

If you have an anthrax, be sure to put on plenty of lemon juice, a powerful antiseptic. This will destroy and neutralize all waste matter, preventing the anthrax germ from burrowing deeper. Keep lemon on it day and night. When one lemon is used up, roll another one, cup it out, and fit it over the anthrax. Have it strapped around with adhesive tape. When the carbuncle is very painful, put on hot applications, alternating with cold, the hot two or three times as long as the cold. That will soon relieve the pain.

Q. What is the cause, cure, and prevention of boils?

A. The human system wants to eliminate all excess waste matter, and it may have to go out by way of boils. The cure is to live on natural foods, which always leave your body in a clean state and never give you waste matter to eliminate. Along with this, it is well to take such baths as will eliminate the impurities nearest the skin, and I recommend sun baths every day between the hours of nine and twelve; also an Epsom salt bath two or three times a week, just before bedtime. Do not use soap. Simply cold sponge off the jelly-like substance which the Epsom salts will have brought out on your skin after ten minutes or so in the water. Bathe ten minutes and rub off, three times. After the final cold sponge, go to bed.

An alternate-day fast, too, is to be recommended. This will take care of the excess mucous being formed. The forces of the body will be permitted, thereby, to concentrate upon the task of waste removal. Protracted, continuous fasts should never be indulged in, for they are dangerous.

Q. How can the pain from boils and carbuncles be reduced? Is lancing necessary?

A. When you have a boil, there is nothing better than to take a little wheat flour and a little raw honey, make a paste of these ingredients, and put it on the boil. Place some absorbent cotton and adhesive tape over it, and leave it there. It will take the pain away. Apply a fresh poultice every day until the boil is gone. Lancing is the wrong way to eliminate a carbuncle or boil. Nature will open it when it is ripe and ready to expel its waste. Cutting spreads it, but honey and flour will make an outlet for the pus and alleviate the pain.

Q. I have been on live food for one month. I now am breaking out with blood boils which are very sore. What should I put on them to draw out the core?

A. I anticipated someone's asking that as I was talk-

ing on that subject, and I have already answered it—
put honey and wheat flour meal over the boils.

BOWELS AND COLON

Q. What are the symptoms of colitis and how can
it be cured?

A. The symptoms? A bloody bowel movement, one
that hurts you and is irregular; a pain up and down
the left side in the region of the descending colon,
though more often on the right side. Frequently colitis
is mistaken for appendicitis. Cure: do not take any
food into the stomach; it would have to be digested
and its contents passed over that sore place. Instead,
feed yourself through the rectum by means of enemas
of cereal water. Strain the cereal before you use it.
Give yourself, also, a daily olive oil rub to nourish you
through the skin, and two doses a day of lemon juice.
If you have much pain, put on some hot applications
for half an hour; this will bring a superabundance of
blood into that area, carrying life and material for
repairs. Colitis, too, is generally associated with fever
and fermentation.

As to the lemon juice, commence with very little,
say a teaspoonful, and gradually increase the amount
until you are able to take as much as a glassful. That
will relieve the inflammation. The process will be aided
by the juices that come from the pancreas and the gall
bladder. These fluids go on through, and when they
find any pus, they neutralize it. Lemon is an enemy to
pus. Do not be afraid to take plenty of lemon and take
it clear. Do this every day. Continue for about ten days

or two weeks if severe. If mild, your trouble will probably be gone in three or four days. The colon will have a chance to heal itself, and when it is healed you will get hungry. Then you may eat. Start first with a leaf of lettuce, to see if the colon is all right.

Now for the enemas. Soak a pound of wheat meal or flaked oats in three quarts of water, shake a few times, and after it has set for two hours pour some of the liquid off, strain it, put into a fountain syringe, and inject. Do this twice a day.

Q. What causes a cyst in the large intestine? How can it be cured?

A. A cyst is like an ulcer. An intestinal cyst is caused by eating pepper and salt and other things that irritate and clog up the membrane of the colon. The little villi there are the absorbers of nutriment from food. It does not take much cooked food to clog them. They lie close together and are possibly six or seven times as long as they are thick. Each has nerves and blood vessels. When these are clogged with cooked starch, it sours there, and inflammation sets in. The way to cure this cyst is to abstain from putting any food into the stomach. Nourish yourself by way of the skin through giving yourself olive oil rubs about three or four times a day. Also take sunbaths. The colon should be washed out once a day with a solution of lemon water, which will soon cleanse the villi, destroy the pus, and heal the inflammation. This lemon water should be flushed by a syringe into the colon, using about three cups of water made strong enough with lemon to taste quite sour. Have it rather warm, too, but do not cook it because that would fix the acid in the lemon. Take it raw, and it will do the work in a few seconds, and change into sugar as well. Do this morning and night.

BREAD

Q. I am one of the new raw fooders and have a desire for bread and butter. I have been eating rye crisp and shredded wheat biscuit with pure coconut butter. Is that all right?

A. If you want to be a live fooder, you should live on uncooked food 100 per cent. Some doctors tell you it is dangerous to start in on raw food all at once. I ask you, "Is it harmful to give the baby its mother's milk all at once?" No, it is not. Do not eat bakers' bread, for that is the staff of death. And do not eat any dairy products, for these cause ferment, and some have salt in them which hardens the arteries. Try our raw bread. We do not approve of any cereal bread whatever, but for those who demand it, we have unfired wheat bread, nut bread, flaxseed, carob, and olive bread. We have these five different kinds of unfired bread on hand at all times.

BREATHING

Q. I have heard that slow breathing aids health. Is that true?

A. Remember, breath is life, so teach every sick person to inhale and exhale slowly. It is the slow breath that does the most good, that oxidizes, that refreshes the lungs. Short, quick breaths are very dangerous. A short, jerky breath will soon kill you. The longest lived animal is the one that takes the longest, slowest breath; that is the cobra. They say he requires twenty minutes to each breath, and that he lives to be from five thousand to ten thousand years old. The longest lived people are the ones who breathe the slowest. Include deep breathing exercises in your "daily dozen."

Be sure you get good air. All outdoor air, no matter how bad it is, whether rainy, damp, or in whatever condition, is always better than indoor air. It is always well when we cannot get the very best air, as in our city life, that we should keep ourselves well supplied with natural foods which can give us the oxygen, nitrogen, and ozone we need for our bodies. It is also wise for all those who live in the city to have an outdoor bed to sleep in, since at night we have far better air than in the daytime. We should have our sleeping quarters away from the congested district—the farther out in the open, the better for you.

BRONCHITIS

Q. Can bronchitis be cured by the raw food diet, and how long would it take?

A. It can be cured, but no one can tell you how long it will take. It depends on many different circumstances; for instance, on how bad your condition is, on how many complications you have. If you have had bronchitis for one year, you will get rid of it more quickly than if you have had it for ten years. Bronchitis is the result of catarrh, and there is only one thing on earth that can cure catarrh; that is, natural, raw food, with its vitamines and organic minerals.

Q. What is the best food for a person laid up with bronchitis?

A. There is no natural food diet that will cure one disease and not another. I have had many a patient who suffered from three or four different diseases at once. I treated for only one, and the food got rid of the others as well. So you see this system is honest and does the work. You really need not inquire about a diet for tuberculosis, bronchitis, inflammation of the stomach, or appendicitis. Eat the natural food that you like best and it will get rid of every single one of these diseases. Mucous-forming, clogging cooked foods caused these conditions. Live fruits and vegetables, properly eaten, destroy mucous—they do not manufacture it. They will purify the blood, thereby nourishing the entire body.

Q. Are hot applications beneficial in the case of bronchitis?

A. Yes, you may use hot water or some onions and potatoes ground up to a pulp and then heated. The heat will help break up the congestion.

BURNS

Q. What is the best remedy for burns?

A. For burns and scalds, get some carron oil, which is nothing but linseed oil and limewater. Soak a cloth in it and lay on the part affected. The pain will stop like magic. Take care to protect the skin, which has a watery serum in it. This serum should never be drawn from any form of blister or burn. Nature provides it to shield the process of healing. Save the blister. Many people think the water has to be drawn out. No, do all you can to protect it. Bandage it so that it will not break; avoid bruises. Never drain it, no matter how large it is.

Should you have a skin burn that does not blister, as for instance a burn from a hot iron, take some baking powder or saleratus at once and make a paste of it. Put on the burn; it will take the fire out immediately. Keep this paste on as long as the injured spot still hurts. In case you are required to dress burns, keep the burned particles under cover without any secondary dressing, so that there is a chance for the air to get to them. When burned so badly that the flesh is cooked, this flesh will have to come off, but do not take it off. Never take the burned particles off with your own fingers, with an instrument, or by any other process. Let Nature cast them off herself. Leave them there until Nature has had a chance to build up new tissue below, a new formation that will cover the veins and arteries underneath and avoid a horrible looking scar. It may take months, but it is worth while.

Keep the burned spot brushed with some pure olive oil applied with a camel's hair brush. You may put into the oil a little lemon juice, but not much. Use this on the burn twice a day, morning and night.

Feed the patient on liquid foods—just liquids, as these are easily assimilated and absorbed. It is most essential to give him the juices rich in blood materials. Try to feed in such a way as to avoid elimination, except enough to get rid of the poisons and thus heal the sore. Fresh air is important in the healing of any burn or any kind of wound. With proper nursing, one can be restored to a natural condition and can avoid scars to a great extent. The trouble with many surgeons is that they tear off that cooked flesh, with ugly scars as a result. Just leave the burned particles untouched, for they will help to protect the under skin, from which the new layer of tissue comes. Everything grows from within outward, never from the outside inward.

If you have a fire burn that is not close to the nose, say on your feet or legs, or on your back, get 4-X ammonia from the drug store and apply it with absorbent cotton. It will do wonderful work: take the fire out, relieve the pain, and start the healing process. Four-X ammonia is extra strong. If you live on natural foods, you have a great advantage over cooked-food eaters, because your blood will be in the very best condition to make repairs; also in the very best condition to keep the injury from going deeper.

CANCER

Q. What can be done to cure a chronic case of cancer?

A. It depends on how old this case is, where the cancer is located, and how deeply seated. A cancer in the neck or head region is truly dangerous. In that case we can only try to steal a march on it, and do not promise anything. Sometimes, if we can give the cancer patient a little hope, it may be that we can neutralize the vibration that eats away the flesh and puts more poison into him. We shall give the person food that feeds the body but not the cancer. The cancer is a scavenger pure and simple, and it cannot exist on living food; it wants waste matter. Therefore, when you have nothing but living food in your body, when nothing but live foods are introduced there, the cancer will suffer. It may be a hard task for you to get used to the new diet, because under those conditions you will probably want cancer food as badly as the cancer does. You may wish that you could eat some cancer food once in a while, just to satisfy your appetite. But do not do it under any circumstances. You must starve that brute. And when the cancer appears to be growing, when you feel the lump is getting larger, good; because in a head or neck cancer those tentacles that went into the head and around the back of the neck cannot find any more food there, and so are drawing in and curling themselves around the body of the cancer. That is the reason why it looks bigger, but do not be discouraged —you have won a real victory.

Cancer is a filth disease, and you should do all you can to keep yourself clean. Wash, wash, wash—Epsom salts baths two or three times a day if you can endure it; fresh air baths and sunshine; sweat baths in the sun with exercise, taking care not to exercise the muscles that are involved in cancer. Keep on, and when you find that the cancer is commencing to loosen in its nest, then you may leap for joy. It is dead, starved to death. What next? Let it rest awhile. The time now has come for Nature to choose in what way the elimination will take place. Do not fear, it will choose rightly. Get plenty of sunshine right over where the dead cancer is, and plenty of Epsom salt baths. Keep clean, as already stated. Soon you may form a boil under the body of the cancer when enough waste mat ter there will have decayed. Then this decayed matter will form a head, and the head work itself out. When it comes the whole cancer goes with it, for the cancer is now loosened from the healthy tissue. When it has all come out, wash the tissues with lemon juice and they will heal. I have never known this method to fail.

There are other kinds of cancers not so easy to get at, but probably much easier to cure—for instance the uterine cancer. We have not lost a case of uterine cancer yet. We have lost one of rectal cancer, the worst kind there is, because in the rectum hard feces pass the cancerous growth and keep irritating it. That is why it is so much more dangerous than the others. But I still believe that this individual who died with cancer of the rectum would have lived if she had had proper nursing.

A cancer patient is very sensitive. Do not let him grieve. Worry kills more cancer patients than anything else.

Q. Has any really valuable research work been done on the cause and cure of cancer?

A. I may quote Assistant United States Surgeon General A. M. Stimson, who makes the dogmatic remark that there is no cure for cancer and no remedy known that will arrest the disease when contracted by a human. Furthermore, "It is hoped through laboratory work that a cure will be discovered, but it will be years before this work will be accomplished. Of course, there is always the possibility of a satisfactory cure being revealed by accident, but that chance is quite re-

mote." Dr. Stimson goes on to say that one of the experiments being conducted by the government employs
osculating current of very high frequency. That will
not cure it. Why? Just because osculating currents
cannot remove filth from the body. Another method
reported by the doctor is one announced at the Inter-
national Congress, whereby one thousand rats were
first artificially infected by cancer, a compound then
developed by laboratory workers, which, when injected into the rat, caused the body cellular activity to
increase and the germs to perish. That is another futile
method of trying to cure the disease and at the same
time leaving the filth in the body.

In this connection we might mention Dr. Drews on
cancer problems. "Cancers and tumors often grow
where the tissues have been injured, internally or externally, by accident, surgery, or hypodermic injections. However, they need a predisposing condition for
their existence and growth. The blood and tissues saturated with proteid waste poison is a predisposing
cause. In ninety cases out of one hundred the trouble
has been traced to flesh foods. The blood which contains the normal quantity of the positive organic salts,
absolutely eliminates the cause and cures or destroys
the disease. The cure consists in abstaining from all
animal foods and all cooked proteid foods, and feeding
on those unfired foods which are rich in organic
sodium, calcium, magnesium, and iron. The herb and
root salads are the most important."

Q. Is sunshine of value in cancer cases?

A. Remember, sunshine is one of the great aids to

health. Yes, it helps to cure external cancer. You may also use a reading glass to direct the sun's rays to any cancer, with great benefit. There is a wonderful curative value in sunshine, plain or intensified.

Q. How shall one treat outside cancer?

A. Put honey on external cancer. Wash off daily. That will cure it if done persistently, together with proper diet and natural living in general. You may also use a poultice made of mashed sheep sorrel. Put the sorrel into a bag, dip into hot water, and put over the wound. After it has healed sufficiently, a hot water compress will do.

Q. A friend has a bleeding cancer in the uterus. If operated, will it spread?

A. It should not be operated upon. She needs all her blood to get well, and the operation will not do her a bit of good, to say the least. No operation that has been performed as yet has ever cured cancer, but only created more cancerous tissue. A cancer is not a local condition. The cancer fastens itself to a certain place, true, but it has really created a home for itself throughout the entire body. It lives on waste matter and creates more waste from the system in order to get food as it grows. Cancers are scavengers, and we can cure them by truly feeding the body, thereby starving the cancer. Eat pure, clean foods; starve the cancer to death, so gradually, however, that it goes to sleep, stops feeding, stops growing, and is finally expelled. Its location in the body makes no difference.

We must stop the bleeding because the good red

corpuscles should remain in the body. Try an absorbent cotton tampon. If that will not stop it, make a tampon of cobwebs. This will stop bleeding instantly, and is absolutely harmless.

Q. Please explain the right way to cure cancer on the liver; also in the intestines.

A. Liver and intestinal cancers send a discharge or waste fluid out of the bowel duct which will often cause irritation and constriction to the extent that the elimination of these fluids will finally become impossible. Cancer is a very treacherous and dangerous disease. It is hard to tell whether it is too late for cure or not, but let us do the best we can. Where there is life, there is hope. This is what we must do: find the fruits the patient likes best. They may be strawberries or fresh pineapple. These are very powerful enemies of the cancer. These will be good morning foods. Flaked nuts may also be taken with them. For the noon meal, you may choose spinach, rich in sodium and chloride, in iron, calcium, magnesium—a wonderful food for purifying the blood. Put some rhubarb juice, as a dressing, on the spinach. Rhubarb is also an enemy of cancer. Take it in liquid form as a beverage or dressing, and not too strong.

As for exercise, do not twist the body or bend, because that will cause friction on the liver. Cancers must be taken unawares, and, if sleeping, kept so, until we have taken all food away from them and they have starved to death. Then the cancerous tissue will separate itself from that great gland, which will gradually be rebuilt with new tissues and will push the cancer right out. It will do that just as fast as it can without rupturing anything. Then, when the cancer has all been eliminated, you will be a well person once more. I have proved all this by many cases in my own practice. One cancer was eliminated in the stool, as a lump the size of a goose egg. The patient will have to endure considerable pain. To quiet this, use hot applications, alternating with ice applications.

Q. How about a chocolate-brown skin cancer? What is the cause?

A. This means an accumulation of mineral crystals in your skin, put there by the blood. This ordinarily begins in middle life and is often incurable. It is, fortunately, not very common. The best method toward a cure is to soften the skin over the hardened growth with a solution of caustic potash. Break up that skin and let it peel off. Then commence to treat with hot applications. The first two or three applications of caustic potash will usually kill the growth, and you will have a chance to destroy it forever by getting new blood into your veins through a more rational way of living.

Q. Can one be cured of a cancer of the face? This party has had it for eight years.

A. Well, I helped drive one out of a man's neck. This patient lived on raw food for a year. Then he applied lemon juice and honey to the cancer, and finally concentrated sun rays through a reading glass, thereby finishing the business.

Q. What is your advice for cancer and depression in the mammary glands?

A. If there is no lump to be felt, merely starve it, but if there is one, you may help by outward applications of sheep sorrel, mashed; of honey; of mashed strawberries; mashed turnip; mashed rhubarb; or cranberries and honey. Choice of these will depend upon which has the best effect on you.

Q. Please give diet for cancer patient.

A. The principal vegetables and fruits valuable here are those in the Rumex family; namely, sour dock, sheep sorrel, English sorrel, rhubarb; also cranberries, tomatoes, oranges, and strawberries. Horseradish and other radishes are good, too. Peanuts are also valuable. They are rich in organic salts, potassium, especially. and also rich in protein. Watercress is fairly good. It will strengthen the lower bowels and the lower organs in general. Strawberries and rhubarb rank especially high in the Rumex qualities. One lady cured her cancer on orange juice; a man cured his largely on horseradish. Mix your horseradish with flaked raw peanuts, half and half. If the cancer is down near the bladder, have the patient eat three ounces of watercress, four ounces of lettuce, and three ounces of flaked peanuts, together. Pineapple is also a first-rate remedy for cancer.

Q. Do you advise radium treatment for cancer?

A. When the radium treatment was first discovered, it was assumed that now at last relief was here for the many sufferers from cancer, but, alas, the victims of this dreadful disease increased in number, rather than decreased. The treatment is very expensive—medical doctors must live in fine homes and drive fine cars, and the radium treatment is one of the methods which helps them to get these things. This does not assume that doctors are necessarily racketeers; merely that the public is being victimized.

CANNED FOOD

Q. Do you advise drinking canned juices of tomatoes, pineapple, grapefruit, grapes, etc.? Are canned vegetables ever uncooked?

A. The answer to both of these questions is "No." All canned and bottled fruit and vegetable juices, as well as all canned foods, undergo processing by heat or by the addition of preservatives or preservative processes in some form or other. If this were not the case, fermentation would begin immediately. Juice your own tomatoes, or, better yet, eat the fruits and vegetables in their natural state. If your system cannot handle all the pulp, expectorate it. So-called "cold packs," where the cans or glass containers are treated by steam or boiling water, certainly cannot, by any stretch of the imagination, be said to be a natural process and preserve for us the original vigor of the foods. Neither can treatment of juices by sunlight or artificial rays be considered a natural process. In Nature, the juice is never found separated from the pulp cells which contain it. Once it is exposed to the air and light, immediate deterioration takes place. No system of extracting juice can prevent air from touching the juice at some point or other in the process.

CATARRH

Q. Please tell me how to treat a case of chronic catarrh.

A. This disease comes from a constant use of dairy products, which are phlegm-producing foods. Cheese, butter, buttermilk, sweet milk, and whey are all fermentable. They produce phlegm and lay the foundation of all catarrhal conditions. Furthermore, the phlegm covers up the mucous membranes and makes them foul. It weakens the system, until you become sluggish. Then watch out for constipation, indigestion, and appendicitis, all secondary results of catarrh. There is catarrh of the bowels, of the bladder, of the liver, of the stomach, and of many of the finer organs of the system, not only that of the nose and throat. You will find it in every part of the body, though it may be localized in the stomach and the bowels long before you detect it in the throat.

It can be easily cured, for any kind of live food that you like will do it. The best combination is no combination. Try your food mono-diet style. Try an apple. If one does not satisfy your hunger, eat another, or a dozen, if you want them. Just so with oranges. Eat one or a dozen, but eat them alone. If you mix or blend them, provided they are all raw (nothing cooked), you will find them absolutely wholesome, absolutely health building, but you will build health faster and be more cheerful if you go on a mono diet.

When you live right on natural food you can never keep catarrh. You will spit and cough, but keep on. The mucous will, and should, all come out. You will probably pass stringy phlegm from the bowels. You cannot get it all out even in three or four months. It may take a year or two.

Q. Kindly tell me how to cure a catarrhal condition. Muccus forms in my throat, but I do not have a cough.

A. A catarrhal condition in a young person is easily relieved, but in a grown person the tissues have already been coated with many layers of phlegm, perhaps as many as you are years of age. Eat nothing but live food. Try taking deep breaths, and hold, so that the air in your lungs will force the blood up into the head. Notice, you will have coughing and spitting spells, a process of elimination. Keep on. You will suffer at first, as Nature will break down some more phlegm, which you will thereupon cough and sneeze out. It may take a year or two, perhaps even five years, before you are rid of your catarrh. You will have a crisis every three months, or every six months, and thus keep on eliminating until your catarrh is entirely gone. This is the way Nature works to get it out of your system. You can help this process along in different ways: sniffing mint leaves is good; also try lemon juice to clean out the nostrils, and gargle the throat with it. Swallow a little of the juice, too.

Stop taking dairy products or anything cooked. Keep away from salt, vinegar, and sugar. Live on roots, herbs, and a little fruit each day, the fruits in the morning; but keep mainly on tuberous foods, like turnips, potatoes, carrots, etc. Choose the one you like the best. That will clean out your digestive tract quickest of all. It will not be long before your head will begin

to feel better. When you eat potatoes, carrots, or turnips, do not chew them fine; leave little lumps. These
will aid the stomach to tear up all the phlegm. This
will work loose, and the food will carry it along
through the pylorus and the duodenum into twenty-five
feet of intestines and the colon; then you are rid of it.
The phlegm may soon stop dropping. If it does, keep
on with the régime until your system is devoid of mucous. Sometimes, however, as I have previously remarked, it may take more than a year to do that. I
know individuals who lived faithfully on this food for
eighteen months, and even as long as two years, before
they finally got rid of the phlegm.

Q. Would it be a disadvantage for one having
catarrh to live at the seashore? Would it be too damp?

A. Catarrh is always aggravated by a damp atmosphere, but the dampness will help you bring out the
poisonous material. The salt water air near the ocean
will help you get rid of it. A higher altitude makes
you feel better, but that does not bring the mucous out
of your system. Get down where you feel the worst.
That is the place to go for a genuine cure.

Q. Would you advise one who has catarrh to discontinue the use of uncooked grains? Are they mucous
or acid forming?

A. Grains are a starvation diet for humans, whose
digestive tracts are not equipped by nature to handle
these starchy seeds. Birds thrive on grain because it is
their natural food. In case of need, human life can be
sustained on them even in their cooked or baked form.

Why try to drag yourself through a keyhole, however, when you may walk in through the door? Nature has provided us with innumerable luscious fruits and easily digested vegetables, which are infinitely superior to all grains. Grains contain starch in large quantity. Raw starches, as well as the cooked, are acid forming, and should be avoided especially by those with a tendency toward catarrh. Acid means mucous—where you find the one, as a general rule you find the other.

CHANGE OF LIFE

Q. How should a woman care for herself during the menopause or change of life period? What kinds of foods are best to eat?

A. A woman, during this period, should always be obedient to her tastebuds. Remember, the tastebuds are your master builders, and whatever food you crave is your food. Eat just enough to get along on, and get plenty of rest.

Q. What can a woman in change of life do for hot flashes?

A. Epsom salt baths are very good to help open the pores of the skin and thereby get the waste matter out. Use, also, fresh fruit and vegetable juices every day. These juices should be taken between meals, at intervals of about two hours, if you like, but not with other food, and up to a half hour before your meal. Fruit juices should be taken in the morning until noon; in the afternoon, vegetable juices, such as celery and pineapple.

Q. Does a woman who has lived on live food and close to Nature experience a troublesome change of life period?

A. Nature provides for those who obey her laws a painless transition from one stage of existence to another. Death itself will become a falling to sleep rather than a painful wrenching away. How much more will the minor transitions be free from even petty annoyances? It is true that to be thus wholly immune from pain, you must live one hundred per cent naturally. That, for most of us, is, under present conditions, impossible. However, we can minimize and practically eliminate the discomfort attendant upon the cessation of menstrual action in woman. Since Nature has provided that the mother should watch over her child until at least the age of maturity, such a cessation of sexual activity as change of life may logically be posited at somewhere around thirty years before the close of the individual's earthly existence. With animals and plants the period is much shorter and therefore relatively inconspicuous.

Q. Will a fleshless diet relieve the distress felt during the menopause?

A. I know of a case where terrible pains during this period were permanently relieved by the elimination of meat from the diet. Meat is highly acid forming; hence its constant use often adds the proverbial straw to the camel's back, even in cases where only a very little is eaten.

CIRCULATION

Q. What is the cure for cold hands and feet?

A. Take plenty of warming foods, such as garlic, horseradish and other radishes, chile, peppers, watercress, mustard greens, nasturtium leaves, dates, figs, and avocado. Combine oil, honey, and starch. Oil and starch are fuels; honey is the match. The three combined, as in olive oil, bananas, and honey, are wonderfully warming. Sometimes just a few figs, or a combination of figs and nuts, or dates and nuts, will warm your blood.

For immediate relief, thrust the members into hot water; or take a shingle and slap the soles or palms hard; or put your feet into ice water. Take them out, rub dry, run around the floor ten minutes, and see how quickly they react. In a cold climate, run around the block barefooted in snow; then bathe the feet in cold water, wipe them dry, and go to bed. A hot bath gives only temporary relief. If you take a hot bath, finish with a cold one, and take it so cold that even cold air will make you feel warm.

As to horseradish, do not take it clear, but grate it and sprinkle a little on your herb and root salads, just so that the taste comes out snappily, tickles your tongue a bit. Or, put some flaked peanuts on it, as much of the peanuts as there is horseradish.

You must be very fond of oranges, apples, and tomatoes, especially oranges, lemons, grapefruit, and all citrus fruits. They cool rather than warm, the blood, and thus are good foods for summer and fall but not for the colder months. You need not eliminate them entirely from your diet; merely cut down on their use.

Q. My legs, from the knees down, feel cold. What can I do for them?

A. Stimulate the blood circulation, and nothing is better for that than exercise. Warm your blood by eating plenty of naturally stimulating food, like horse-radish or peppers. Also encourage the blood circulation in your legs by taking alternate hot and cold baths. Combine all this with deep breathing and sunbaths.

Q. What is the best food to produce heat, energy, and endurance?

A. There are many foods that produce these, but I shall give you the caloric values and then allow you to make your own choice. Oats contain the highest percentage of calories of any cereal. Corn comes next, and so on down the line until we get to the nuts. Dates rank higher than some of the nuts. They are rich in carbohydrates. Protein and carbohydrates are sources of energy. The carob bean is very rich in both, containing from forty-five to fifty per cent sugar and twenty-four per cent protein. It is the protein that makes for endurance, vegetable protein being found in the chlorophyll.

Q. A woman, 43, has a hard lump in the stomach and several in the small intestines. She is usually paralyzed during the night, especially toward morning, so that part of the time she is compelled to sit up. She has lived on raw foods for about four or five months without any apparent improvement. What would you advise?

A. If she has lived 100 per cent on live food, her blood is probably much improved, but she seems not to have been able to get the blood into the paralyzed muscles. There are artifiical methods of getting the blood there: you can move the afflicted parts with your hands, or produce a hyperemia by putting on a hot water bottle, or pad, or hot brick. This heat will draw the blood into the tissues. Try a little massage. The muscles will absorb the blood and become stronger. Raw food may be eaten, and yet it may be impossible for the blood to get to the muscles in question until it is helped along with sunshine, deep breathing, and copious sleep. Sometimes you see dumb animals stretch, roll, and jump. Why? Because they feel an impulse to replenish some nerve or muscle. Some of us are far too dead as yet to get that impulse, but when you have lived for several years on these foods, you will now and then feel the urge to a do a little stretching, or make other movements. Try it. Don't resist.

Q. When I awake in the morning, my hands are asleep. What should I do?

A. Stop lying on your hands. When you go to sleep, be sure that your arms are free. Lie in such a way that your body is not resting on your arms—then the blood will circulate. The blood pressure is not as strong at night as in waking hours, for the heart skips every other beat. Therefore it does not take much to make an arm or hands numb.

Q. I have a numb feeling in my arm every day. What causes it?

A. Take some strenuous exercises, such as running, or handball, that will induce your blood to circulate quickly. Your arm gets numb because the heart does not beat fast enough.

Q. What is the cause of numbness in the shoulder, or lack of circulation in the arms and hands when asleep at night?

A. You must be lying in such a position as to cramp some nerve that leads to the arms. Try lying on your chest with your face down. Take your pillow away. To stimulate circulation, there is nothing better than exercises. Take the daily dozen not only once, but a dozen times, and see if it does not help.

Q. What is the cause of jumps and jerks in my leg when I get cold in bed? There is no pain.

A. Poor circulation. Take a good warm bath and finish with a cold shower. Then take a little exercise, and you will soon be rid of your trouble.

Q. Will you tell us something about how to build up health where there is low blood pressure, slow heart beat, where one chills easily and has sluggish blood circulation?

A. If you have been living on natural food for any length of time, it is quite easy to stimulate your blood circulation and warm your body by exercise. A live fooder can get warm readily by very little exercise, but for one who does not live on raw food, it requires quite an effort. Right breathing is important. Fill your lungs full of air, slowly; then hold your breath, clasp your hands together, and swing back and forth a few times. The moment you let go, all the blood vessels quickly resume circulation, as the exercise has given them a start.

CIRCUMCISION

Q. Is circumcision necessary?

A. Not nowadays, as a rule. Sometimes one finds an adhesive formation on a baby, and it may be possible to avoid cutting it by massaging it out. Sometimes a small snipper or fine scissors will do the work. A little careful minor surgery will not do any harm. Do not hurry things, and, above all, maintain perfect cleanliness. Never allow such a delicate organ to accumulate filth. We are told that Abraham, in ancient days, commanded that all male infants be circumcised, but it was merely because the Hebrews knew no other way to combat venereal disease and sexual abuse.

CLOTHING

Q. Are clothes necessary to health?

A. Going without clothes, or very few, will give you better health, stimulate skin activity, give you energy from the sun, brown your skin, and give you dynamic force. There is nothing better to make healthy blood than the sun shining on your skin, and when you get live food in your stomach and then let the sun shine on you, it is doubly good. Abbreviated bathing suits! What a blessing, what a grand chance we are giving the sun to shine on our backs! — not for the sake of merely wearing less clothes, but for the sake of getting the

benefit of the sun into the blood! I would like to see
every man, woman, and child wear one. Clothing is
not an index of true modesty. In fact often those who
would measure our morality by the comparative skin
area covered by cloth, may be more interested in divi-
dends than in virtue. Many of our California beaches
now permit boys and men to go about in shorts only.
Take advantage of this wonderful opportunity to get
sunshine and stimulating air directly on the skin.

Q. I have been ridiculed for not wearing a coat and
hat. What is your viewpoint?

A. Wearing hats is absolutely unnatural even for
women. All clothing is unnecessary. I do not approve
of the wearing of hats, especially tight ones. Women
will soon be as bald as men if they do not stop wearing
tight turbans. If you must wear a hat, get a loose-fitting
one. When you buy a straw hat, never buy a stiff-
brimmed one, but one which will yield in the crown.
Go bareheaded whenever you can, as sunshine is a
valuable tonic for the scalp. As for going coatless, I
would advise it whenever it is feasible. You will not,
in our modern society, always find it so, however.

Q. What material is best to wear next to the skin
—cotton or silk?

A. One is made by the silkworm; the other is grown
in the field. Does not that give you a hint? Consider
too, how you make up the material. If the cloth should
be loosely woven, or even a mere net with threads about
an eighth of an inch apart, then you will get sunshine
and the air will touch you. White, or unbleached ma-

terials, are the best for clothes which come in contact
with the skin. One eliminates contamination from dyes,
besides having a cooler garment in summer, since the
sun's rays are reflected, not absorbed, as is the case
with dark shades. White or unbleached linen or cotton has still another advantage over darker colors;
that is, it makes for cleanliness, as one has to wash it
more frequently.

COD LIVER OIL

Q. Is cod liver oil a raw product, and do you recommend it as a medicine?

A. All animal and fish fats are rendered by heat,
while olive oil is obtainable in a cold-pressed state.
You cannot cold press animal oil, but you can do this
to olives, nuts, or any other natural vegetable food, because there is nothing in these latter to hinder the oil's
escaping. Cod liver oil is a fish oil and merely pollutes
the system. It therefore should not be used. Get your
vitamines from live, wholesome foods, and from the
sunshine.

COLDS

Q. I have had a cold for more than two months
now. How can I get over it?

A. A cold results from the presence of waste matter in the body. What is commonly called a cold is the
process of eliminating this waste, largely through the
nostrils. Had you not been clogged with waste matter, you would never have put Nature to this extra job
of house cleaning, that brings with it a characteristic

soreness, hoarseness, sneezing, spitting, and general exodus of phlegm. Do not be alarmed. When Nature has finished, you will scarcely recognize your body for its bright, new "feel." Do not try to obstruct Nature by checking the cold. Rather aid her efforts by drinking lemon juice, eating bulky, coarse salads, and by getting plenty of rest.

Why should we humans catch cold any more than a rabbit does, or a squirrel, or a gopher? We pamper our bodies by wearing heavy clothes that make us tender as a house-plant, and consequently subject to periodic colds. If we did not wear any clothes, we would not be slaves to temperature changes, because our skin would soon learn to perform its natural function of thermostat for the body, the pores opening in warmth, and closing in chilly weather. In all events, we should wear as few clothes, and as simple ones, as possible.

As to cure, take only liquids for a couple of days. Stop eating solids until the phlegm has come out. Take hot water and honey, or hot water with garlic and honey.

COLIC

Q. Is there any food particularly good for colic patients?

A. First in order comes the tomato; second choice, the cucumber. Both are excellent remedies and contain a high percentage of health-building qualities. Eat the one you yourself prefer.

CONSTIPATION

Q. Please tell me what causes constipation. I have been on live food for some time but am still constipated.

A. Constipation is caused by eating cooked, refined mushes, where there is no roughage, and at the same time plenty of salt, all heated so that your stomach will not rebel while eating. There is no strength-giving energy in cooked foods. Consequently, sooner or later the bowels must get weak. With a chronic lack of roughage to exercise your internal muscles, you lose peristaltic action. Some people, moreover, say they have been on live food for four or five years and are still constipated, but you will find that they are occasionally eating some cooked food. Do not make that mistake. When you are on raw food, eat nothing but 100 per cent raw food—fruits, herbs, and roots. Only then may you claim to be a true live-fooder.

Now for the treatment of constipation: at night, put a tablespoonful of flaxseed into a glass of water and let it stand all night. In the morning, one half hour before breakfast, stir this up and swallow, seeds, water, and all. Do not chew the seeds; swallow whole. These seeds have a jelly-like consistency that lubricates. One-half hour later your stomach will be ready for breakfast. Now eat the fruit you like best, not chewing it over-fine. In fact, swallow it as coarse as you can and as fast as you can, just as though you wanted to catch an express train. But mix it well with saliva. Then, after the meal, eat all the dried olives you can. The olives are rich in oil, protein, and roughage. Do that every morning. Now at noon, the herbs—always the ones you like best, possibly lettuce, or celery, or spinach. Chop up coarsely. Eat from about seven ounces to a pound of the chosen herb. If you have a big appetite, well and good, but do not chew your food thoroughly. Moisten it with saliva and gulp it down; work your tongue instead of your teeth. Then dried olives again. And do not forget to soak the flaxseed to be taken before your evening meal. A half hour before the evening meal, take this, and for supper about seven ounces to a pound of grated carrots and an ounce of honey, mixed, together with three ounces of flaked peanuts. Do not chew this too much, either.

If, after following these directions to the letter, you do not have a good bowel movement on the second or third day, I do not know my business. This will force you to have a movement, and in absolutely the most natural way. One of the reasons you do not have bowel action is because the bowels are empty, because you eat food, which, by the time it gets to the stomach, is practically liquid, and by the time it gets to the intestines, is almost totally absorbed, with no roughage left.

Q. Some years ago I had an operation for lung trouble, without gaining relief from constipation. I am a beginner on live food and your advice as to what kind of food I should eat and what habits I should adopt. will be appreciated.

A. The first thing to do when you wake up in the morning is to raise your arms over your head, spread your fingers, and twist your body. Then do the deep breathing exercises—put hands up above the head and inhale, bring them back to the side and exhale. Do this seven times. When you bring your hands up, your lungs are stretched lengthwise. Then put your arms out in front of you, swing them backward and outward, inhaling as you do so. This stretches the lungs sidewise. Thus you can oxidize the blood that has circulated very slowly while you were asleep. After you have done these exercises, start the abdominal movement: lie on your back, bring the knees up, and work the muscles of the abdomen in and out. Do this until you are tired. Rest until the tired feeling is gone, and then do it again until tired a second time. That will be all the exercise necessary until the next morning.

After you have gotten up, drink a glass of orange juice. An hour later you may have breakfast of your choice of fruits, and, after this, try three ounces of some flaked nut that you like, such as almonds or Brazil nuts. They must be flaked, because, if not, they will be out of harmony with your fruit. If you do not want to flake them, eat them two hours before the meal. Then eat a dozen dried olives, or four or five pieces of olive bread. You should not drink anything for two hours after the meal. During the forenoon, you may drink fruit or vegetable juices or water, up to one half hour before the noon meal. Here, take your choice of the herbs. If you like lettuce, pull off the outside leaves, put on honey, roll up like candy, and eat. Next try two or three ounces of flaked peanuts and another dozen dried olives. During the afternoon you may drink rhubarb or pineapple juice at intervals, to within half an hour of supper time. Your evening meal should consist of roots. If you like carrots, you may eat them whole. You may dip them into a little honey if you care to. Then eat some more olives or olive bread, and I dare say that before the week is up you will have plenty of bowel movements. You may find the olives bitter at first. But you may be glad to know that bitter food makes good muscle. It also induces the activity of the peristaltic tissues and is an aid to digestion.

Action will possibly be slow. Patience, then, and perhaps an enema, may be necessary. Should you miss one day in bowel action, take an enema, using a syringe and cool water. That should start it, but if it does not, wait until the next day and run another cupful of water. I do not usually recommend this, but since you have been living unnaturally for so long a time, we must sometimes resort to unnatural methods to bring you back to a natural condition.

Q. Are three daily bowel evacuations necessary to health?

A. You will have a call shortly after every meal if you are in a normal condition and thoroughly cleansed. Be obedient to that call. If you have but one movement a day, decomposition will have begun to take place in your colon, producing gas. Ordinarily, the bowels of a cooked fooder do not move at all by peristaltic muscular action, but by mechanical means; that is, by gas pressure. It will take some time for you to remove the phlegm coating from your colon and bowels to make the natural movement possible, but do not be discouraged; you will win out. Natural food is digested in from two to three hours, whereas cooked food digests in from five to six hours. By eating natural foods, you

will give your stomach and digestive tract one or two
hours more rest than if you indulged in cooked food,
and thus you will keep the peristaltic muscles in first-
class condition and be free from constipation. Then,
too, no cooked foods are laxative, but all raw foods are,
by their very nature. As an aid to establishing regular
bowel movements, make an effort immediately after
every meal, even though you may not be successful for
the first week or two. You can thus help Nature in
forming the beneficial habit. When it is once fully
formed, no muscle in your rectal organs will be powerful enough to prevent the bowels from having a movement, so strong will the urge be. You will actually be
forced into line with Nature's law.

Q. Is all live food laxative? My constipation seems
to be worse now that I am on live foods.

A. Sometimes laxative foods seem to cause constipation. You may have eaten cooked food so long that
you have lost the natural peristaltic movements of the
bowels. In that case, gas has replaced them, gas caused
by the fermentation of food in the bowels. When you
take natural food, the fermentation stops, there is no
gas, and the bowels do not move. What are you going
to do, go back to canned foods? No, give yourself
enemas, temporarily; eat your food coarse so as to
force your bowels to work. If you suffer from griping
during this process, roll your bowels with your hands.
That forces the obstruction on. Repeat if necessary. It
will relieve pain instantly and you will soon have a
natural bowel movement.

Q. Please give directions for taking flaxseed and olives for relieving constipation.

A. Flaxseed is absolutely harmless. It is a lubricant and a producer of mechanical action in the bowels. Stir into a glass of water a tablespoonful of it. Let it stand all night. In the morning, stir again, and while the seeds are floating, drink, seeds and all. Do not chew the seeds—swallow them whole. The little points on each seed get into the corners of your bowels. These seeds, too, give off a jelly that gets into the waste matter coating the lining between the villi. It will break the refuse up and clean the bowels slick as a whistle. You may take flaxseed for a week and not notice much difference. Consequently you may have to have an enema for a starter, but keep on with the flaxseed three times a day, a half hour before each meal. Prepare another glass immediately after you drink one, so as to have it ready for the next time.

As to the olives, eat them whole if you can. If you do not like them that way, pit, grind fine, and mix with your fruit salad in the morning, with your leafy salad at noon, and the root salad at night. Eat as many as you can after each meal.

Q. What is "agar"?

A. It is an Oriental seaweed, which, when eaten, swells up twice its size and gives you mechanical bowel action. Use agar in place of gelatin in your desserts.

Q. Is olive oil good for breakfast to clean out the intestines, and how much should one use?

A. You may use olive oil on the fruit you eat, about

a tablespoonful at a time. It is perhaps better to take your olive oil in the form of dried olives. Why not take flaxseed before meals and dried olives after? That will help the bowels.

Q. Is the avocado a good laxative?

A. That depends on your general condition. If you like avocados, eat them. They are very oily, fatty, and therefore will lubricate, but, remember, do not chew them thoroughly, rather as coarse as you can. Mix well with saliva. It is bulk that gives the laxative property. If you do not like this particular fruit, leave it alone. You will not be benefited by eating avocados just because they are fatty, and therefore laxative.

CONTAGIOUS DISEASES

Q. What is the cause and cure of smallpox?

A. We get smallpox because we are full of waste matter, on which smallpox scavengers feed. These generally start in the stomach, breeding in the intes-tines. The cleaner the body, the freer it is from disease. Do not be alarmed about so-called contagious diseases, for once you are clean physically there is no contagion as far as you are concerned. No disease will then be able to attack you, for the simple reason that there is no waste matter to feed on. When there is no food for the scavengers, the bacteria will starve to death.

Smallpox can be eradicated within three days if everyone will do what I say. Never be vaccinated for smallpox—it is more dangerous than the disease. If any of you go into a community where smallpox signs have been put up, drink a glass of fresh cider, tomato juice, or citrus fruit juice every day, and I guarantee that contagion will not touch you. Live on natural live foods, of course. You will not only build your health every day of your life, but keep yourself immune from every pestilence. Anyone who has already contracted smallpox should drink a glass of orange juice each day, and the skin should be washed with lemon juice. Give plenty of olive oil rubs, too, and you will clean up that case of smallpox quicker than any doctor ever did. Besides that, you should get rid of all filth that may be on the body, bathing daily.

Q. Can diphtheria be cured by live food?

A. Diphtheria is a contagious disease of children. We very seldom hear of an older person coming down with it. No child can have diphtheria unless it has a predisposed condition in its body, waste matter that forms a basis for the propagation of the germs. Diphtheria is a peculiar scabby formation over the membrane, or part of the membrane, of the throat. Medical doctors mostly use, or used, innoculation to overcome it. Nature never intended that anything should be put through the skin with a needle. Nature never intended that anything which was good for the system should go by any other routes than through the digestive tract, by external application, or by bathing.

The first discovery of a partial cure for diphtheria was made by a woman of South Carolina. I was only a boy when this event occurred. My father was studying the question quite seriously, and he learned about a case of diphtheria that had been cured there by an ordinary washwoman who was handy with different household remedies. She had used kerosene, a few drops in sugar, had dissolved the whole mess in a cupful of warm milk, and given it to the child, with good results. While it was not the really natural way, yet it seemed to kill the bacillus, and the child got well. Today we use a different remedy. There is nothing better than lemon, honey, and warm water, together with hot and cold applications around the throat. Only a few doses of this are needed to eliminate the worst forms of diphtheria, and if a child takes the remedy in the beginning, at the stage of incipiency, it will never fully develop the disease at all.

Q. Are children fed on 100 per cent live food and no milk or raw eggs, immune from measles, diphtheria, and the like?

A. Yes, provided they have lived a one hundred per cent natural life. Natural food is extremely important, but, after all, not the whole story. There must be sunshine, fresh air, the minimum of clothing, exercise, sleep, normal home conditions, and a fair heredity, before such a guarantee can be met in its full sense. For all practical purposes, however, such a child will be immune from contagious diseases and may safely go anywhere without fear of harm.

Q. Why does an occasional parent contract whooping cough, which is supposed to be a disease of childhood?

A. Such so-called children's diseases are not confined to children in all cases, only as the usual thing.

Grown-ups, however, when they do contract a disease of this kind, suffer acutely from the elimination that a child can handle without too much trouble. Children's diseases are acute and violent, and the parent's body is not as resilient or vital as that of a child. Hence the difference in their reaction. In both the adult and youngster, however, it is poisonous waste matter that is being eliminated. The need for such elimination should not exist in either of them, and is the signal of maladjustment to the laws of life.

Q. Is black death still a common disease?

A. When I was in Panama, I visited three different cases of black death, the plague they dread so down there. Black death is really a tropical affliction, since the cold air of the north seems to destroy the germs. In tropical countries, coconuts are plentiful and very good. I got the patients I mentioned to drink coconut milk in quantities, and they got well. This got the health officers of the hospitals interested, and now coconut milk is used for the cure of bubonic plague and black death.

Q. How should a bad case of measles with high fever be treated in a child six years of age?

A. Only a child who has been living wrongly is susceptible to measles. The first stage, characterized usually by hoarseness and phlegm in the throat, should be treated with lemon juice sweetened with honey, diluted about 50-50. This should be drunk by the patient three times a day. In addition, put an onion poultice made of boiled onions over the chest. This will have a two-fold effect—the inhaled onion fumes will be beneficial, and the inflammation will be drawn out from the bronchial tubes, thereby easing the elimination and bringing about a recovery. The poultice should be renewed each day, and the entire body, with the exception of the poultice-covered chest, sponged with lemon juice. Plenty of fresh air should always be admitted into the room, and during the second stage, when the rash appears, the room should be darkened. During convalescence there is generally an intermittent fever. Apply hot or cold towels, as desired by the child, mainly in the region of the spine and trunk. When measles is treated in this manner, the patient will recover rapidly.

Q. What can be done for a child three years old that has whooping cough? It has eaten much raw food for about a year, and sometimes milk and cooked food.

A. When you say it has been fed milk and cooked food, you yourself point out both the cause and the remedy. Improper living has brought the cough— proper living will remove it when the process of cleansing is completed. Do not think particularly about stopping the cough, but rather about how you can aid in easing the flow of phlegm from the system. The child is expelling mucous collected in the course of improper eating and perhaps in other details of living. Put hot and cold applications on the neck, alternately. When the neck is full of collected blood, have the child do some neck exercises—up and down, as nodding; from side to side; circular-rotary movements, and what not. All of these will aid in promoting better circulation in the neck, at the same time loosening the phlegm. Honey is good in such cases also—a few spoonfuls alone, in warm water, or in fruit juice.

As to contagion, if your child is full of mucous, it will be susceptible to the whooping cough germs emitted by those having the disease. If it is clean internally and externally, there is no danger.

COURTSHIP AND MARRIAGE

Q. In courtship, is it considered natural, ever, for the woman to take the lead?

A. I think it is more nearly right for the woman to find the man than for the man the woman, for the woman has a finer instinct for the one she desires.

Q. What would be the right way of sex mating in order to be in harmony with Nature?

A. Too many of us do not understand how to choose mates in the present status of society. Too many eat so much flesh food that they are excited with passion instead of love. That is why there is so much bloodshed, hate, and inharmony in family life. There is no bearing and forbearing between parties to the union. We must always remember that we are not perfect in the present state, and also that we are going to attain to a higher degree of perfection. If you have a mate who is willing to live in the same environment as you, you have a wonderful jewel.

CRAMPS

Q. Sometimes I have foot or leg cramps after retiring, and the feet and legs may become rigid. What can I do for it?

A. Take the leg between the hands and twist it. The pain will stop immediately. The next thing to do is to put hot applications on the cramped spot. That will bring the blood there in abundance and satisfy the aching nerve. Give rubbing treatments and hot applications every night, and you will soon get rid of your pains. Commence to correct your diet immediately.

Q. What is the cause of cramps, and what is the remedy?

A. Get the poisons out of your system. The nerves will not complain until they have to. Get up a perspiration in the sunshine. Do not take a blanket sweat or a steam sweat, but take it in the sunshine, by exercise, if feasible.

Q. What causes cramps in the stomach? How should they be dealt with?

A. Often, stomach cramps are due to sudden changes in bodily temperature, as after the eating of ice cream or the drinking of ice water, with a hot meal. The best remedy is to drink a hot lemonade and apply hot towels to the stomach.

DEAFNESS

Q. Will this system of eating help bad hearing?

A. Yes, it will help total deafness if the ear drums

are unimpaired. I have seen people totally deaf for twenty-five years, cured, their hearing restored. One old lady, after a fairly long course of treatment with no apparent improvement, suddenly one morning heard a canary bird sing. Her hearing came back like a shot. That is the way it comes, as a rule. Those afflicted seem to be deaf as a stone until the very last moment. Then a peculiar adjustment takes place—you scarcely know what. This woman was bewildered, went around looking up and down, finally saw the bird, and knew that she was hearing again.

Q. Can defective hearing be overcome by correct diet? If so, how?

A. Defective hearing is the result of eating cooked foods, dairy products, and devitalized material of all kinds. You have filled yourself with so much phlegm and have weakened your system so that it cannot discharge this phlegm. It crawls into the Eustachian tubes and makes you hard of hearing. All deafness where the eardrums are not ruptured, is due to catarrh. All those who want to get well and have perfect hearing, must live according to Nature.

Try this exercise for deafness: take a deep breath through the mouth while holding the nose with the hand, and try to blow the breath out through the nose. Take the hand away, and then swallow. Also, you might try putting your hands over the side of the head, palms over the ears. Push tightly, then take the hands away suddenly. You can hasten recovery by taking a drop of spirits of camphor on a tuft of cotton and putting it into your ear before you go to bed at night. Camphor will neutralize the irritated condition. Do not pour it into your ears, however. In the morning you may have a queer feeling and have to cough or sneeze.

DIABETES

Q. Please give the symptoms of diabetes.

A. Fever, a great appetite, and an intense craving for sweets.

Q. What is the proper diet for one troubled with diabetes?

A. You must avoid commercial sugar, cooked sweets, milk, cheese, butter and eggs, fish, as well as all forms of animal flesh. You may eat natural greens, fresh fruits, vegetables and roots, all uncooked. You may use oil and honey in moderation, if you like them, but not too much at any one meal. You can always satisfy your exaggerated craving for sweets by eating the right kind of base; for instance, some flaked walnuts or almonds with your morning fruit. The best base for the leafy vegetables you should eat at noon, is the raw Spanish peanut. When you eat leafy vegetables alone, they are easily assimilated, and you soon get hungry again, but if you eat the flaked peanuts and honey, they will keep you until evening. Then, with your evening roots, take peanuts again, with honey, and your stomach will be satisfied until morning. With the fruit breakfast have flaked almonds or other tree nuts. Try living this way for a time, and you will soon not know yourself. Eat no cooked food whatever. People who eat two raw meals and one cooked

and the like per day, are not making much headway.
Pure honey will not create unnatural sugar. Many
diabetic cases have been given honey and have gotten
well. People in Los Angeles who were given up to die
by the most expensive doctors have been cured in this
way.

Q. What fruits and vegetables are most beneficial
in diabetes? May nuts and olive oil be used?

A. Yes, and also honey. Remember to eat always
such fruits and vegetables as you like best. You may
have to change occasionally. Diabetic people are very
fickle in their tastes—every now and then they must
have something different. Be sure to find that food
which seems most delicious. Keep away from bakery-
starch breads. Eat cereals, but eat them raw. There are
many different kinds of bakery products made for diabetic patients, all a total failure. Diabetes cannot be
cured that way. You must have live food, not garbage.

Q. Of what use is the giving of insulin to diabetics?

A. Insulin is given to diabetics because the normal
production of insulin by the pancreas has partially or
completely ceased. As long as this insulin is adminis-
tered to the patient, he will feel much better, but that
does not stimulate the lagging organ to begin producing insulin again of its own account. Quite the contrary; it is weakened. There may be justification for
giving the patient insulin in critical periods when he is
still unable to receive it from its natural source in sufficient quantity. The basic necessity, however, is to get

the pancreatic gland functioning normally. This can be done only by restoring it to its natural vigor. To do this, you must live according to the laws of Nature.

DIARRHEA

Q. What raw foods would be beneficial in a case of diarrhea?

A. All natural live foods are laxative. They work as an eliminator. They can be compared in result with massage. Give yourself a ten minute massage over the bowels, kneading them, commencing on the right side, up the ascending colon, across the transverse colon, and down on the other side. Continue for ten minutes with both hands. Knead the bowels first on one side and then on the other. This, strangely enough, is the way to help get rid both of the condition of diarrhea and that of constipation. The diarrhea massage, however, should generally be less active than that given for constipation.

As to food, take that which you like the best. It was at one time generally believed that blackberries were good for diarrhea. That was because of their eliminative effect, but we now know that all live food works in that manner. If you have diarrhea, it may be due to a fever in the bowels. There is very likely something irritating you there. That is very easy to cure. Lean back over a table—hands behind to balance—as far as you can. Do that two or three times and you will probably be all right. What has been accomplished? When part of your intestinal lobes are inflamed and you in this way stretch yourself upward, you will change that

peristaltic movement. You may thus be able to dislodge the substance that is causing the diarrhea, and
make it pass on and out. If it does, you will have no
more trouble.

Q. What is the cause of dysentery?

A. It may be due to excessive elimination by way
of the bowels. If you are eating eliminative food in
quantity, go on an alternate-day fast for a short while.
You will find the trouble clearing up rapidly, sometimes even magically. Temporarily, stop eating roughage foods, such as cabbage, lettuce, beets, etc. These
sweep the intestines vigorously, which is, for the time
being, precisely what you do not want. After the fast,
you may eat them cautiously, in small quantities.

DIET

Q. You say that people should eat only the fruits
which grow in the locality where they live. Should
people, then, who live in the north, eat citrus fruits?

A. Are you now living on cooked foods or are you
living on California-grown fruits and vegetables? If
you came here, say, from New York, you must not
continue eating your customary New York food. You
must get the foods grown in California. Foods grown
here have the same vibration as the California climate.
If you live in that way on raw foods, you will never
get sick again.

In the northern states we grow potatoes, wheat, oats,
barley, rye, flax, carrots, turnips, rutabagas, cabbage,
apples, and the like. They are all good food and are

grown and enjoyed in all climates. On the other hand, oranges for the northerner are not good. They do not grow except under semi-tropical and tropical conditions. They prepare the blood for living in warmer climates. They have a tendency to thin the blood, and cold climates demand a rather thick consistency of the life fluid. All citrus fruits show this tendency. In colder climates you need more roots and hardy vegetables. The cabbage of the north is much heavier and hardier than the cabbage that grows in California. People who want to eat tropical fruits in the north will have to take the consequences. It is all right to live that way during the summer months, but even then not as beneficial as eating them in the climate where they were grown.

Q. Please inform me if it is true that raw food is harder to digest than cooked food.

A. I shall let you judge for yourself. It takes from two to three hours at the longest to digest live food, whereas cooked foods require up to six and eight hours to digest even partially.

Q. Leafy vegetables do not seem to satisfy me; neither do root vegetables when taken alone, or even with honey and nuts.

A. You probably are not eating a sufficient quantity. Some people require only one meal a day, others four to six. Perhaps you are one of the latter type. If one helping of vegetables or roots does not satisfy you, take two, or three, until you have had sufficient. You may eat some more of the same food an hour or two after your meal. Remember, peanuts are always permissable with roots and vegetables. The peanut is not as easily digested or assimilated as these foods and will stay by you until meal time comes around again, if you eat a sufficient quantity.

Q. Is a cup of raw peanuts too much at a meal?

A. If you eat nothing else, no. But if you do, it will probably be too much. It depends on the size of your stomach and how big, physically, you are. Some people will take a cupful; others will be satisfied with one or two ounces. Most of you will eat less when you get normalized, but now you are still actually starved.

Q. What should a workingman eat, and how much? Do you recommend cereals?

A. A workingman should eat just as much as his stomach seems to desire, and when the desire is satisfied, he should stop. Of the several different kinds of starches, choose the one which is most delicious to you —it may be wheat, oats, corn, a fruit starch, a nut starch, or starch from bananas, or it may be the starch from cabbage. One doing heavy work should add to his morning fruits two or three ounces of flaked nuts, at least. They will maintain him for four hours, until noon. Then he may mix lettuce and peanuts together to keep him until evening, when he may mix the peanuts with roots. The peanuts should also be flaked.

Cereals are really bird food, but what will give tissue to the bird will also give tissue to man. We make an oatmeal pemiken; wheat meal, with raisins and figs; and cornmeal pemiken, mixed together with nuts, oil, and honey. Any one of these makes a tasty breakfast food. These pemikens may also do for a noon meal In the evening, you should make yourself a nice vegetable salad.

Q. I do not find the fruit breakfast in itself sufficient to last me until noon. Can a grain which has been soaked by water be combined with a fresh fruit breakfast?

A. No. But you may take some flaked nuts with any of the fruits. They will satisfy your hunger until noon. Nuts go very congenially with fruits. The only way you should take wheat or oats with fruits is with dried fruits, like raisins, figs, and dates. You may grind them together and let them blend for two or three days. Then eat them. This is food for hard-working men, not for people of leisure. Another thing, you must expect some gas formation, because all cereals will produce ferment, but since it is raw cereal, it will produce a sweet ferment. The sweet ferment, true, is offensive, but the sour ferment that comes from cooked food and dairy products is both dangerous and offensive.

Q. What can a workingman carry for a healthful lunch?

A. Try an orange, apple, peach, some apricots, some of our pemiken. Include also a cup of flaked nuts, with honey, and perhaps fruit juice to drink. Always make your lunch of whatever you like best—that is important.

Q. Are two pounds of raw fruit or raw vegetables too much for an elderly man's meal? Nothing else is eaten, except possibly a tablespoonful of ground nuts.

A. I want to ask you a question. After you have eaten two pounds of fruit (and I hope you eat this in the morning), are you hungry? If not, then you have had enough. I shall ask another question. After you have eaten two pounds of vegetables, are you hungry? If not, you have eaten enough. If you find that the food you have eaten gratifies you and is satisfying, well done —you need no more nor less. You will know if you have had too much—by an uncomfortable, heavy feeling.

Q. What is the system of diet you recommend?

A. Why not follow this program: fruits in the morning, with a few flaked nuts; herbs at noon, with some flaked peanuts; and in the evening, roots, again with flaked peanuts? Fruits in the morning are your eye-openers. You are just getting out of bed, you have had your shower or a cold, stimulating bath, but you want something in the stomach, something to help eliminate waste matter which has accumulated during the night's sleep. The fruits are the best eliminators and the best tonic. Fruits are golden in the morning, silver at noon, and lead at night, so do not eat fruits at night, as a rule. There may be certain anatomical conditions which might cause fruit to be better at night than in the morning, but that is exceptional.

The leafy herbs are very good at noon. They grow in the sunshine. The sun kisses them and gives them their chlorophyll and vitality. They will keep you well until evening.

In the evening you will want something to help repair your body while you are asleep. What type of food will do this? The roots that grow in darkness, under the ground, that see no sun, but are rich in earth salts because the edible portion grows in the soil itself. When you eat them at six P. M., by nine they are all digested. You then go to sleep, and the digested roots commence to do their building. Is not that in harmony with Nature?

I recommend peanuts because they are congenial with all forms of leafy vegetables and roots, and because they are so stable and nourishing that you can work for three or four hours without getting hungry. The trouble with most workers who live on live food is that they eat too light foods, which are assimilated so quickly that hunger comes long before the time for the next meal.

Q. Is it correct to eat fruit just before going to bed, or, say, two hours after eating at night?

A. If you are well and you feel like eating the fruit, you may do so, but you are beginning or are in the grip of a bad habit. Fruits are not night foods. They should be eaten in the morning, because they are an eye-opener, a tonic, the eliminators of waste that has been produced in your body during sleep. The daylight foods are leafy herbs, like lettuce, cabbage, cauliflower, cresses, celery, and endive. These are grown in the light of the sun. We do not eat their roots, just the tops. These are very good for tissue building. They make you strong, healthy, and robust, as they are rich in earth salts. You should always eat the kind you like best. It is well to mix a few peanuts with these leaves. In the evening, eat those foods which grow in darkness, the roots. They will also do your repairing in the darkness while you are asleep. This system of eating is in harmony with the vibrations of the earth. Do this, and you will know how it feels to be really happy.

Q. What foods are mucous forming?

A. All cooked foods, for these digest by fermentation; also, some foods that produce fermentation although they are not cooked, such as milk, butter, cheese, and eggs. If you want foods that will never ferment, try roots, or herbs that grow close to the surface of the earth, excepting only onions, garlic, and leek. Be careful about mixtures, too. The best combination is no combination. The mono-diet is the best diet for every living animal on earth, humans included.

Q. Is it well for a person to eat two kinds of food for breakfast?

A. Yes, two kinds are permissible, particularly if you are well. If you are not well, eat naturally; that is, eat one kind of food at a time, not two or more. You may find this difficult at first, but the results will make the effort worth while. Do not eat an orange, then an apple, then a pear, and a half dozen figs. Eat one thing only, taking as much of it as you find necessary to satisfy you. When you are satisfied, wait until you get hungry again, and see what your tastebuds will call for.

Q. Which is the better breakfast: oranges and nuts, or oranges and prunes?

A. Oranges and nuts. If you want prunes, do not

mix with oranges. Eat them separately. Eat oranges and flaked nuts or prunes and flaked nuts. Now the food which is best for you will taste most delicious. If you find that prunes taste better than oranges, then you need prunes, for the time being, rather than oranges, but if you like oranges better, then you need oranges. You need not worry about calories, or about minerals and carbohydrates. Your tastebuds never make a mistake.

Q. Please give your opinion of the no-breakfast plan.

A. Very good, for those who have easy jobs; for instance, bankers, bookkeepers, and others who work with their brain and not with their hands. But a laborer with a shovel or axe; a blacksmith; a carpenter; or a farmer who walks all day in soft soil, into which he sinks a couple of inches at every step—such men need three good, substantial meals a day.

Q. What is the normal food capacity of the stomach?

A. That depends upon the nature of your occupation. If you are doing desk work indoors, your stomach will not want much food, and this food may be of a kind that is easily assimilated. But if you are a worker who has to swing hard with a pick and shovel all day long, your body uses up much muscular energy, causing your stomach to demand plenty of food. You will, in this case, eat two or three times as much as the banker. Since you use more muscular power and energy, you need more material to replenish it. Cooked foods often bring about enlargement of the stomach, especially with a hard-working man, for he craves the right kind of reconstruction material and finds scarcely any in all the quantity he can possibly eat. Cooked foods have scarcely any building power and cannot give you good blood.

Q. Can one overwork the digestive tract and kidneys by eating great quantities of fruit? I like fruit and eat different varieties from breakfast until two P.M., and then eat some salad about six.

A. If you feel no distress after meals of this kind, there will be no harm done. Keep on until you grow tired of it.

Q. Are nuts, peanuts, and honey considered part of a mono-diet when they are eaten with a fruit or vegetable, or should they be eaten at a separate meal?

A. A mono-diet means that you eat one article only. It means to eat fruit *or* almonds, not fruit *and* almonds. A mono-diet helps one to get well quickly. A person on this diet will, as a rule, not be one doing heavy physical or mental labor. As for such a one, he is usually not satisfied, especially at first, with such a radical change in his habits, and hunger will set in within a short time. When you are sick, follow the mono-diet one hundred per cent and let no cooked food interfere with your progress.

Q. Is it right to eat only one kind of food every day, or is it best to have a variety?

A. It is well to change, but change only when Nature calls for it. For instance, if you like apples, keep on eating them every morning as long as you want to, but when you feel you are getting tired of apples, find some other fruit. It is not necessary to make a change every day. Change only when you are tired of what you are eating. If the food does not taste up to par, it will not do you much good, but when it tastes delicious, it will.

Q. I live on raw food and find I have not the strength in lifting I formerly had. What is lacking in my diet? I use many nuts, and peanuts.

A. You may use too much concentrated basic food. You may need more fruits and vegetables, something for elimination as well as reconstruction. You need fruit in the morning in sufficient quantities to give you the power of elimination. If you were perfectly clean and purified, you would not have that weak feeling. You must get all of the impurities out of you. Only then, when they are all out, will you commence to reconstruct muscular tissue, for natural food will not build or add strength or muscle if there is anything broken down in the way.

Always have your nuts flaked if you are eating them with other food. If you eat them whole, wait until two hours after a meal, because with the meal they will not assimilate and will cause indigestion; but flaked, they will mix and digest harmoniously.

Q. How much lemon juice do you advise a person to take with his daily food?

A. You may take as much as your tastebuds desire, even to the extent of half a dozen lemons. It will never injure you to eat anything in the way of natural roots, vegetables, or fruits to the extent of your capacity. Some people can enjoy eating one orange and have a good after effect. Another person could enjoy eating it too, but with bad after effects. If this distress has been marked with one orange, then do not eat two the next time, but rather half an orange. Keep on with the oranges because they are doing good work, cleaning and purifying, perhaps even taking cancer out of the system. Eat only such amounts as you can endure. That applies to all foods, not merely oranges.

Q. I crave apples, yet they seem to disagree with me. What shall I do?

A. When you are hungry, consult your tastebuds. Go get some fruit and taste it. If it does not taste as it should, try something else. When you find something that appeals to you as delicious, that is the food you need. If you eat it and it distresses you badly, that means the food has really hit the spot. You should eat it, but not too much at any one time, for all natural food is live food and will twist the stomach out of shape if you take an overdose. When you find something that tastes good, for instance an apple or watermelon, take one mouthful every morning until you feel that there is no distress after you eat it. Finish your meal, however, on something that does not distress you. Soon there will be no more trouble with the single mouthful. Then take two mouthfuls, the next time three, then four, and soon you will be able to make an entire meal of it. What is it doing? It is getting you well. When you find any natural food your tastebuds call for, and it distresses you, you will know that you have found your best friend. Take it within the endurance of your power of retaining it.

If you are not distressed at all from any natural foods you are eating, then it is hard to tell when you will get well, as disease tissue is often covered over with a thick catarrhal coating. It sometimes requires five to six years, but keep on. Remember, there is reconstruction going on all the time, and when your body gets rebuilt, regardless of your age, you will become immune from disease. The older you are, the longer it will require. Your circulation is not as lively as it once was, but stick to it. Do not get discouraged. This is the best and only means of getting right with God and Nature. We know from experience—and experience is the best of teachers—that there is no better way of eliminating disease than directly through the bloodstream.

Q. Why does eating any one of the following foods put my teeth on edge so much that I cannot eat anything else for hours: cherries, oranges, apples, French dressing, plums? I have been living on raw food nearly a year.

A. Do you eat raw foods one hundred per cent, or mixed with cooked? We have a few half and half raw fooders, who say they live one hundred per cent but eat bread, potatoes, and other cooked things. This will not do, because the one forms an acid and the other tries to get you well. You are attempting to shake hands with God and the devil at the same time. Your condition will be overcome by living entirely on natural foods. Do not drink when you are eating; only between meals—up to one-half before and two hours after—and you will soon find there is a change for the better.

Q. I have an aunt who has suffered from cancer. Would it be safe for her to go on a one hundred per cent raw food diet all at once? My mother has rheumatism in her legs. Would it be safe for her?

A. The safest and easiest method for anyone who desires to start living on natural foods is to drop cooked foods at once and permanently. Yes, give them all the natural food they care for. There may be a little of what seems unfavorable reaction at first. This merely means that the nourishment is acting as a medicine. It is killing the bodily poisons in a large way. They may think they cannot endure it, but they can. When it seems to hurt badly, smaller amounts should be taken, until the body is accustomed to the new source of nourishment; but have them keep on with the same food, just as before.

Many people from the East have said, "When I get to California, I'm going to eat lots of oranges." What happens? In a week they break out in a rash. Many such have come to me for advice, and I invariably tell them to keep right on eating oranges. They think it queer, but the oranges will get all the poisons out of their bodies and will finally make them immune from disease.

Just so with any cancerous condition. You may happen to hit upon some food that is particularly delicious to you; that, for you, will be the prize-winner. A man I know had two cancers. He liked horseradish root and could eat it as you would carrots. He carried horseradishes about in his pocket and ate them by the mouthfuls. What did they do? They cured his cancers. In five months they had completely disappeared.

Q. Can green alfalfa be used as a salad, to eliminate a gaseous condition of the stomach and bowels?

A. Yes, it may be used, and it is a non-ferment. If you like it, eat it. You will get some mineral elements in alfalfa that you will not get in many other things, but it is not necessary to eat alfalfa unless you really care for it. Do not eat anything because someone tells you to do so. Judge by your tastebuds. They are the master builders. Consult them. Because alfalfa contains certain elements lacking in most foods, or because it has long roots, is no sign you should eat it. Your body may not want those elements. It may prefer cabbage, or lettuce, or spinach. Do not judge by a table of mineral contents. That is a mistake. Consult your tastes, your idiosyncrasies. That gets results.

Q. What are the warming foods for one who suffers from cold a good deal?

A. There are quite a few warming foods. Dates are delicious and a splendid warmer. Eat a pound a day, provided you like them, and see if you do not get warm. If you do not like them, find another food that will do the work—for instance, horseradish, the common radish, mustard greens, nasturtium, and watercress; also honey, oil, nuts, peanuts, raisins, or dried figs. When you get cold, you can help matters along with physical exercises. Swing your hands back and forth a few minutes and see how quickly your body warms up.

Q. Is the use of saccharine in place of cane and beet sugars ever advisable?

A. It is an inorganic coal tar product, and not a live sugar. The only organic sugar we can get in pure form is in comb honey.

Q. Is the cocoa bean good to eat?

A. It is, after you have taken the bromine out of it, but that costs more than the bean is worth.

Q. Is French dressing good to use on root salads?

A. Yes, as long as you make it sour with rhubarb juice instead of lemon juice. Then it would be all right. If you use a French dressing on fruits, employ lemon.

Q. Does heat below the boiling point harm vegetables, cereals, and fruits? If so, how?

A. Soups, fruit juices, and the like, if made from uncooked herbs, vegetables, and fruits, may be heated to blood temperature, or slightly over, without damage, but never to the boiling point.

Q. If one cannot eat honey, will sorghum do?

A. No, absolutely not. Eat figs and dates, but not sorghum. It is prepared by cooking.

Q. Is there any value in cooked fruits or vegetables?

A. Yes, they serve as bulk to dilate the organs.

Q. From what vegetables or fruit do we get the most chlorophyll?

A. Beets, for one, probably the best source; second, spinach. Figs and prunes also contain a goodly quantity of chlorophyll. Beet tops are equal to spinach in this respect.

DIET FOR CHILDREN

Q. Please tell me what you consider the best diet for children twelve, thirteen, and sixteen years of age. They eat live foods, but they look undernourished and pale. Should the mother feed them on grains, nuts, and dried fruit more often?

A. No. The grains are objectionable. They are not human food. Your children have no gizzard, as they do not belong to the bird family. Therefore they are not able properly to digest cereals or whole grain. Your children may eat what fruit they like best in the morning, the herbs at noon, roots at night. For red cheeks and the look of being well nourished, give the children plenty of greens and fruits. Be sure there is a little honey to go with them, and some olives after each meal, to aid the digestion. After the child has eaten these foods for some time, the blood will contain the proper building material. Remember, the master builders, the tastebuds, are the guide to good blood. Whatever your children like best is what they need. Do not think you should give them more iron, or potassium, or this and that, in forms which children dislike. Give the child, as the adult, that which is most delicious to its taste, in all cases.

When well saturated with live foods, the child should take especial care to go nude in the sunshine between ten and eleven o'clock each morning, or in the middle of the afternoon. It ought to get the sun on its skin some time during the day, and those are the best hours. Sunshine will invigorate and stimulate the blood action and the blood cells. This will give the child an inexhaustible fund of energy and of good blood. Strength will come with this régime.

DIET FOR INFANTS

Q. What is the best food for children before and after the weaning age?

A. When a mother cannot give the child her own milk, and cannot find a wet nurse, then she should feed it on diluted fruit juices. Those which the mother likes best will usually suit the child. The only milk you should use in that case is milk made from almonds, peanuts, or coconuts, derived from the nut butters and finely ground coconut. You may add a little honey to these milks if you wish. The nut milks, then, should be baby's food until it has teeth, when you can give it other things, like spinach juice and cabbage juice; but do not give it any animal milk after it has been weaned, for it loses its thymus gland when eighteen months old, and cannot digest milk without creating phlegm and catarrh. The fruit and vegetable juices mentioned are rich in lime, which is needed for creating bone during this period of rapid growth. The banana and avocado may also be used, but do not give them full strength. Dilute them; they are too strong for the child. The avocado is a wonderful fruit for baby because it contains only two per cent protein. Carrot juice is also excellent. Do not imagine that the baby cannot adapt itself to natural foods—it can, and will flourish.

Each of us is equipped to use mother's milk from the time we are born until we are, at the latest, eighteen months old. I have known a mother to nurse her child until it was four years old, not because the child needed it, but because she liked to nurse. She had acquired an unnatural habit. These cases, fortunately, are few and far between. More, nowadays, do not want to nurse children at all; they make bottle babies of them instead. Any woman who intends to give birth to a child should prepare herself to nurse it as soon as it is born. If she does not do so, she should not have children. She is unnatural. Most babies are weaned, in fact, wean themselves, in eighteen months' time. Long before you commence to wean the baby, start feeding it some of the natural fruits, and herbs, and roots. If you do this, the child will soon wean itself. It will just forget milk—that is Nature's way. Everything in Nature comes easily. Disease can never attack the child successfully if you raise it on natural foods. It is impossible for the child to be sick if you care for it correctly.

Q. Should an infant be fed only at regular hours?

A. The baby will soon be able to indicate when it wants food if its instinct has not been spoiled. When baby is hungry, it will first try to let you know by a pleasing method. Then, if food is not forthcoming, it will try something not quite so welcome. Still unsatisfied, it will get displeased, and then you will hear plenty of squalling. A baby should not be forced into a fit of crying before its wants are attended to. That is bad both for the child and for the mother. If the mother has not sufficient milk, it would be well for her to eat more lettuce and spinach. These very often increase the flow of milk. In the meantime, give the baby some diluted fruit juices. Do not cook anything for the baby. In general, the hours of feeding are best regu· lated by the baby itself, for adults may want to over· feed it, overload its little stomach, or unwittingly starve it, while the baby will never make those mistakes.

Q. Should a newly-born baby be kept without food for two or three days?

A. When a child cries, it should have nourishment. What you mention is a mistake. It is unnatural. As soon as a baby is born and it opens its eyes and is washed, the stimulation of the washing, as well as the breathing of the child, makes it demand food. The first food should be mother's milk, given without any preliminary drawing out of the fluid. This first milk has in it a substance that will cleanse the child's intestinal tract from a black slimy substance present at birth, and which, if not removed, will make the child constipated from the very outset. Whenever the child cries, thereby giving signs of wanting food, the mother will feel the impulse and desire to hug the offspring to her bosom and give it milk. This impulse should be obeyed, regardless of what people may think. The impulse is precious, and by following it we never make a mistake. It is true that the baby can live for three days or so without suffering for the want of food, but no healthy baby, born of a healthy mother, will ever be without an impulse to take nourishment at least within twenty-six hours after birth.

DIET FOR NURSING MOTHERS

Q. What are a few of the natural foods to cause nursing mothers to have plenty of milk for the baby? Is avocado a good food for her breakfast?

A. Yes, avocado is a very good food, but if the mother does not relish it, then she should forget about it. The finest foods for her are the greens that she likes best—spinach, cabbage, endive, chicory, mustard greens, water cress, etc. Lettuce is very good, too, for creating red blood. All prospective mothers should prepare themselves by eating natural foods throughout the period of pregnancy.

Q. An infant is undernourished from weak mother's milk. What is the cause and cure?

A. Feed the mother the right kind of food and the milk will be nourishing. When you have a suckling baby, do not give the remedy directly to it, but to the mother, and she will relay it to the baby. That is Nature's way. Spinach alone may be sufficient, at least for one meal each day, or have the mother mix some spinach and lettuce, half and half, with some olive oil and honey as a dressing, and perhaps a bit of rhubarb juice.

DIZZINESS

Q. After eating, I feel dizzy, with a dull feeling at the back of my neck. What causes it?

A. Some people mix fruit with vegetables, others, raw fruit and vegetables with nuts, possibly peanuts. In such cases there will be considerable fermentation, which will then attack the nerves leading to the brain, thereby making you dizzy. Mix wheat and fruits, or wheat and vegetables: fermentation will take place immediately. To be sure, these are sweet ferments, not the sour kind. None the less, dizziness will result. Why not eat a mono-diet instead of a mixed diet? Overeating may also cause the symptoms you mention.

Q. Is it harmful to get dizzy from exercise? What causes this condition?

A. Dizziness from exercising is never harmful. Any form of exercise you are not accustomed to may make you dizzy, but if it is not that, you had better consult your stomach and see what it is you are doing to cause gas signals in the brain. It may even be that you are eating something which produces in your stomach considerable alcohol, or chlorine, with consequent intoxicating effect. It makes no difference whether you drink whiskey or beer, or eat unnatural foods—intoxication is derived from varied sources.

DRINKS

Q. Is not a glass of near beer good at meal time? It seems to clear out the phlegm.

A. You should never drink while you are eating. Near beer, however, is preferable to coffee or tea.

Q. Should a live-fooder drink much water?

A. He need not drink any, unless he so chooses. If he gets plenty of juicy fruits and vegetables, he will find that his thirst is quenched by them just as by water. You may, if you wish, dilute extracted juices with water. Some people with sensitive nerves appear to be over-stimulated by drinking pure fruit and vegetable juices, and in their case it would be better to dilute these with an equal amount of water, distilled or otherwise. You sometimes hear that distilled water is dead water. Well water is dead, too, as far as that goes. It comes to life only in the form of watermelon, oranges, or other organic creations. We should not drink so-called "hard" water, full of mineral salts, like calcium, sulphur, potash, for those inorganic crystals help form gall stones and cataracts of the eye. I believe it is a good thing to drink a glass of water now and then.

DROPSY

Q. What treatment do you advise for dropsy caused by kidney and heart trouble?

A. Kidney and heart trouble have never caused dropsy. The kidneys get sick, no doubt, and the heart may get weak, but the real cause is the taking of poor food into your system. Poor food made poor blood, and poor blood made poor heart action. Keep on pumping dirty water continuously, and you will wear out your implement in a short time, which clean water would never do. So with the heart. You have been eating food that has poisoned it with uric acid. This same blood condition ruins your kidneys, and the kidneys fail. The liver must double its work, and you get liver trouble. Then, in fact, you begin to have trouble everywhere.

Dropsy comes, and will creep up the knees to the thigh, then above the hip, and finally into the trunk. There it strikes at the kidneys and bladder. It finally gets to your heart. If the water reaches your heart, you may never get well again. Dropsy is a very deceptive disease. Take care of it as quickly as possible. Eat all the cucumbers, tomatoes, melons, cantaloupe, you want. They will wash out the kidneys and bladder. Eliminate all cooked foods, such as milk, bread, and meat; also salt, sugar, and vinegar. After correcting the diet you will in time be well again.

DRUGS AND DRUG POISONING

Q. What can I do for arsenic poisoning of the stomach caused by taking a solution of arsenic for a skin infection?

A. I would use an intermittent fast. Live for two days on liquids and one day on solids, alternately, for two weeks. Give the stomach a chance to rest, and use absolutely nothing but natural food. "Liquids," in the above case, means fruit juices.

Q. Is the use of quinine harmful?

A. I have walked about in southern cities where ague was plentiful and have seen the unfortunates sitting in corners, in dugouts, on piles of sacks, every-

where, shivering and burning up in turn. Conventional
doctors usually prescribe saline and quinine. Quinine is
a good tooth destroyer. If you want to get rid of your
teeth, continue for a while taking good doses of quinine. Quinine contains mercurial compounds. Quinine
is habit-forming, a dope. People have come to me
while I was in my father's drug store and offered me
their jewels—watches, diamonds—just for a few grains
of quinine.

Q. Can radium poisoning be cured?

A. There is nothing that cannot be cured if there is
enough vitality left to fight, but when there is none, and
no chance of building any, we have lost our hold.

Q. What can be done for painters' lead poisoning?

A. The first symptoms of this condition are nerve
pains. Later the skin turns blue. This latter implies that
the patient is in a bad way. The painter, sometimes in
handling lead, gets some on his hands or another part
of the body. He should wear rubber gloves, or, better
yet, leather gloves, which the lead cannot penetrate.
Getting the lead out of the system is a rather difficult
process. Much patience is required. Horseradish is an
extremely good cleanser in these cases.

Q. Are drugs ever justifiable? Do they ever effect
a cure?

A. Drugs are poisons which the body must, if it is
ever to be normal again, throw off. This requires effort
better used for other purposes. As to whether in extreme emergencies artificial stimulants, for example,

are ever justifiable, is a delicate question. My opinion
is that Nature is a better doctor and nurse, using her
own remedies, than the whole of the medical profession put together. Nature does not have to learn—she
knows and does, if we give her the opportunity. Therefore, I would say that even in cases of high emergency,
only natural remedies should be used.

EARS

Q. I have had a ringing in my ears for the last four
years. What is the cure?

A. Get rid of the catarrh in the Eustachian tubes
by eating live foods. Also practice blowing the nose in
the following manner: hold the nose, breathe in air
through the mouth, and blow into the nose, but do not
let the air out of the mouth or nose until you hear a
clicking in the ears. If you do not hear that quickly, it
means your tubes are clogged up with phlegm. After
this click, you may be temporarily deaf. In that case
drink a glass of water or swallow some saliva, and you
will soon be all right again. Another exercise is to put
the palms of the hands over the ears. Press hands
tightly, then let go quickly. Do you feel the pulling?
That will relieve the condition in your ear. Do this
three or four times every day. Do the blowing exercise
whenever you feel you need to. Clean your ears with
lukewarm water and a little glycerine.

Q. Yellow pus is running from my right ear. Please
give cause and cure.

A. Cause? Eating waste matter. Cure it by abstaining from all things that create pus. Live on live food

and apply such remedies as hot applications, or sun-shine. I took a reading glass not long ago and focused sunlight through it for ten minutes on a polypus in a man's nose. He lost this growth the very next day. The swelling was down, and he commenced to breathe naturally again. Sunshine is the cheapest and best remedy you can get.

Q. My doctor advises a mastoid operation. Is there any way to bring the mastoid bone back to normal without the use of surgery?

A. Yes. If you have a running ear, light-therapy or thermo-therapy (hot and cold applications) will be beneficial. Sunbathe the infected part every day. Eat nothing but live food; thereby you will get rid of the waste matter which has settled in the mastoid region.

EGGS

Q. Please tell me about the use of raw eggs and oils as a dressing or as a food.

A. Do not use eggs. They have a high protein content, as well as much animal albumen. You may use corn oil, pure peanut oil, olive oil, or sesame oil. Lemon juice or rhubarb juice, however, are preferable to oils as dressings. Olives are better than olive oil, and whole raw corn to corn oil, but if you must "dress" your foods, there are no better dressings to recommend.

ELECTROTHERAPY

Q. What is your opinion of electric treatments?

A. It depends on the one who does the work. If a

man does not understand the application of therapeutic electricity, he should keep his hands off, but if he is skilled and understands his work, he may do much good.

ENEMAS AND INTERNAL BATHS

Q. Are internal baths natural?

A. No kind of internal bath or enema is natural, and you will never need one if you will eat properly. Eat natural foods until they have cleaned you out and strengthened you. You will have a lot of bowel action when you first start on live food because your membranes are covered with phlegm, and this must all be cleaned out before normal movements may be expected.

EPILEPSY

Q. What is the best thing to do for an epileptic?

A. There are three principal causes of epilepsy—malnutrition, a chromatic condition, and internal parasites. You may be suffering from malnutrition and toxemia, or have injured some part of your spine or brain through an accident, or you may have tapeworm. With natural food, no parasite or tapeworm can live very long, for the waste the tapeworm lives on will be cleaned away. In the case of the accident, the bruise or injury has not healed correctly because of poor blood, with acidosis consequently affecting that weak point.

The convulsive attack in epilepsy is mostly due to your body's being filled with so much toxic waste that the nerves get cramped into an unnatural position, especially the sensory nerve and the ones nearest the brain. A person who is subject to such fits never knows when he will have an attack. When he does have one, he generally falls down, kicks and squirms, and sometimes lies on his back, pounding the earth, frothing at the mouth. He appears in terrible agony, but he is unconscious all the while.

Here are two quick remedies. One is to put a cold wet cloth over the face; the other, holding the patient in an upright position—which it will possibly take two or three men to do, because he will be very strong in that convulsive condition—and pounding him on the first, second and third dorsal vertebrae. This will start the heart going more rapidly, and he will commence to revive. When you have no chance to get water, this is the next best remedy.

I had a case in Minneapolis of a woman who had been afflicted with epilepsy for seven years before I became acquainted with her. She had been taken to a famous clinic down state, also to the greatest nerve specialist in the Northwest. All said they could do nothing for her, that she would outgrow it. She was just a child at the time. But years went by, and the girl steadily became worse instead of better. Her two attacks per week at the beginning had increased to fifteen or twenty a day. When she came to me, she was so weak that in order to maintain herself in an upright position she had to hold on to a chair. I found she had a predisposing blood condition, due to acidosis, and, besides, an injury of the spinal cord caused by striking, in a fall, the end of her spine on a steel couch. I wrote out a special diet of live food for her, including peaches, apricots, and pears. There were daily light exercises, and, before retiring, sitz-baths to bring blood into the injured spinal region, followed by a rub-down and bed. In six weeks she had improved tremendously, and soon her epileptic fits left, never to return.

EXERCISE

Q. May a middle-aged man living upon live food indulge in fast running without harmful results?

A. It would be very beneficial. To be sure, if you are not accustomed to it, you should be careful not to overdo. Cultivate your muscles as well as your brain. Start out by a short run every day, and gradually work up toward longer ones.

Q. What morning exercises do you recommend?

A. I recommend, besides the ordinary setting-up movements, a number of bed exercises: first stretch and twist the whole body several times. Then inhale, raising the hands up high over the head in so doing, seven times. That pulls the ribs up and lengthens the lung or thoracic cavity. Stretch your arms sidewise and inhale in so doing, seven times. This broadens the thoracic cavity. Then come the abdominal movements. Lie on your back with knees up and hands at side. When the knees are up, you relax the abdominal muscles. Start working these in and out until you get tired. Then rest a moment and do it again. This last named exercise is especially good to restore abdominal muscles to their original power.

Q. Is there any time when exercise is not beneficial?

A. The patient himself should be the judge in many instances. When, however, there is a feverish condition present, exercise should be minimized, or eliminated entirely, in spite of any desire on the part of the sufferer.

Q. How can one strengthen one's arm muscles?

A. You will have to set up resistance of some sort, weight lifting and manipulation of stubborn forces, such as in an exercising machine. Arm muscles will not be developed unless there is need for their use in daily activity. Therefore, these exercises must be done not once, twice, or three times a week, but every day, and preferably until the muscles get tired. You do not need any elaborate equipment. Go out into the back yard and start piling up the rocks which may have accumulated there. Activity in the out-of-doors is always preferable to that taken indoors. Dumb-bells are fine for this purpose, if you have them.

EYES

Q. Can you give us a remedy for inflamed and weak eyes?

A. Put hot and cold applications over them. Prepare two containers, one with hot and one with cold water, and two small towels, so that you can use one immediately after the other. First put on the hot one, then the cold, but only half as long; the hot one again, and the cold, three times. The purpose of the cold application is to prevent congestion. This process will bring blood to those inflamed or weak nerves. Also give your eyes a rest whenever you can. In the morning, too, put hot and cold applications on your neck, three times hot and three times cold, the hot twice as long as the cold; and do the seven neck movements. These movements will stimulate the many different nerves contained in the neck, and cause them to do their duty to the eyes and the whole cranium. Be sure that you eat 100 per cent natural foods. Prepare them as plainly as possible, and eat only until you satisfy your hunger. Never drink with your meals.

Q. How would you treat a bad case of eyestrain of long standing?

A. Do eye exercises for about twenty minutes to half an hour every day. Then I would give my eyes a slow massage with the palms. Next, I would put my palms over my eyes, and if I saw black, all right, but if I saw other colors I would know that something was wrong, the eye not giving proper interpretation to the mind. The right color is black. When you see green, red, and other colors, your vision is abnormal. The way to cure this is to get a blackboard, look at it, and think "black." Put your palms up over your eyes and think "black." Do this a number of times every day and your darkness reaction will soon be black. When you have accomplished this, you will find another abnormality to correct; namely, power of vision. For this, do some sun gazing. First look through your fingers at the sun. After you get accustomed to that, try looking directly at the sun as long as you can. At first tears will come, but try again. The eyes will soon get used to it.

Do this between nine and eleven in the morning. A few glances should do at first. The time may later be lengthened to suit.

Q. A number of years ago I was looking at the eclipse of the sun, and ever since then the sun keeps dancing in my night eye. It even persists at times in my day eye.

A. Gaze at the sun a little every day. Keep your hands on each side of your eyes so that the rays of the sun will not strike them squarely, and you will be able to look at the sun quite a time before tears come. Keep on doing this every day between the hours of nine and eleven o'clock, and your trouble will disappear.

Q. Should the eyes be shaded in the sunshine?

A. That depends on the condition of the eyes. If you wear glasses, it is best to take them off in walking toward the sun. A visor is needed by some people, especially those who wear glasses, as it keeps the glare of the glass from going into the eye. Some people are not able to take off their glasses, being near-sighted. If you do not wear glasses, I would answer your question in the negative.

Q. Why do black spots float before my eyes? How can I get rid of them?

A. Live on natural foods until the blood is replenished, and then you can expect the vitreous fluid of the eyes to have been replenished also. You may then practice sun gazing, with palms over the eyes at first, but do not attempt this until you have lived on natural foods from six months to a year. Use the palms to protect the eyes so that you will let only part of the sunshine in at a time. Also practice seeing and thinking black, first with the eyes closed, or palms over them. Your condition may be caused by indigestion. For this, eat dried olives after every meal.

Q. Dark clouds float in front of my eyes. Can it be a cataract I am suffering from?

A. It may be due to your feet. I have had a patient who was totally blind, and I had to treat his feet to restore his sight. He could see within six weeks after I started, well enough so that he could read and write. Eat natural foods 100 per cent to get good blood. Give yourself an eye-cupping with olive oil. Also bathe your feet thoroughly every night before you go to bed.

When the man mentioned above came to me, I carefully checked over his physical anatomy and found that his feet were deformed; also, that they sent out a not very wholesome exudation. I took it upon myself to treat his feet, ordering him to wash them twice a day for a considerable time in hot water, then to rub off with a cold towel and walk on tiptoe so as to straighten the deformity in the feet—this every night for a certain length of time. He soon commenced to feel much better, and before long he said: "I can see a little, doctor. I can almost see whether it is a man or a woman I am looking at." Finally he was able to read the printed page again.

Q. Color blindness—what is it and what can be done for it?

A. Your optic nerve sees things rightly, but your mental interpretation of that which your optic nerve sees through the camera of the eye is not rightly made. Practice seeing and thinking black, first with eyes open and then with eyes closed, and practice seeing and thinking other colors, like green, blue, and yellow, until you can readily distinguish one from another.

Q. If the lubricating fluid ceases and the eye gets irritated, what can be done?

A. When the lachrymal glands go dry, in the first place stop eating salt and sugar. And if you are a smoker, stop smoking, since nicotine helps to dry out your glands. Eat such foods as are richest in fluids, say okra, every day, also fresh sweet corn as it comes from the field. Eat all the sweet corn you can. Put hot applications over the eyes, alternating with cold, really hot and really cold, three times each. Then exercise them. Do this every morning and evening. Rub gently with a soft cloth, also. This will help stimulate the lachrymal glands to activity. The exercise mentioned consists in rotating the eye, with your back toward the light.

Q. My left eye waters and is hard to open in the morning, although I am on natural foods one hundred per cent. This has troubled me for years. What is your advice?

A. This is perhaps the result of errors in your past life. Saline substance or other sodium deposit has accumulated there and is hard to get rid of. A few very delicate tubules form the ducts for the tear glands, the tears being a very fine and very clear fluid serving as a lubricant for the ball of the eye. When there is the slightest irritation, conscious or unconscious, it may cause a surplus amount of this fluid to drench the eye It may also be that a foreign substance is lodged somewhere in the delicate tissue. Use hot and cold water applications alternately.

Q. Is it possible to cure cataract of the eye?

A. Y-e-s. That sounds dubious, doesn't it? It seems so merely because the process is necessarily a very slow one and most people do not have patience enough to follow through. Eat natural food. That will help bring the vitreous fluid into better condition and change the peculiar condition of the eye lens. Make a wash of part Epsom salt and part burned table salt. Take one tablespoonful of table salt and brown it in an open flame. Then mix with two tablespoonfuls of Epsom salt; dissolve in seven ounces of clean rain water. Put that into your eye with an eye dropper. Also, once a day give yourself a friction bath just over your upper nerve center. Eat caraway seed in salads, as it is especially beneficial to the optic nerve.

Q. Can anything be done for blindness, except operation?

A. For certain cases, wash the eye with olive oil every morning and night. The olive oil has a tendency to soften the membrane. At the end of five weeks, change this olive oil bath to scraped decomposed apple. Scrape an apple and let it decompose in the air until it gets brown. Then put over the eye like a poultice.

Q. Can we diagnose disease by observing the eye?

A. The eye is a barometer of bodily conditions. It will indicate when there is anything wrong with any part of the body. If there is a marking in the white outside the iris, just across horizontally from the pupil, there is something wrong in the chest. If you find any marking in the circle around the pupil, there is without doubt some trouble in the stomach. If you have any marks above the pupil, you will find something wrong with your neck, head, or eyes, and there are signs by which you can know whether it is in the cerebrum, cerebellum, nose, or ears. Iriodiagnosis is especially valuable in detecting the presence of inorganic mineral deposits in the body. See the chart of Dr. Allen of Chicago; also Dr. J. Haskell Kritzer's book, "Iriodiagnosis."

A. Does the color of the eye give a clue to one's health?

Q. I know of a case where a greenish-grey iris became bright blue after several years of living on natural foods. Waste matter accumulates in the iris as well as in other parts of the body, indicating its presence by a dark discoloration. The skin becomes clear when the bloodstream is purified. Why not the iris? The greenish-yellow tint in brown eyes often disappears after a prolonged period of natural living.

Q. Do you advise the use of glasses to help impaired sight?

A. In certain cases glasses may be necessary temporarily. Do not, however, neglect corrective exercises, diet, etc., which will bring them to the point where these crutches are no longer required. If your eyes trouble you without the glasses, you will have to bear with this device for a time. Oculists, as a rule, supply only the crutch—you will have to supply the intelligence. However, you may be lucky enough to find an oculist who is also a naturalist. In that case he will advise you in detail, depending upon your individual case.

FAINTING SPELLS

Q. Please tell us what to do when someone is found unconscious.

A. The first thing to do is to put your ear to the patient's heart. If you find a vibration there, which, though not like a beat, is a murmer or a kind of trembling, there is hope. Lean the individual up against your chest, put your hand on his forehead, and commence to give him concussions over the first, second, and third vertebrae, which have control of the heart action. A pulsation will soon take place. Next, if possible, give him a swallow of cold water—just one swallow. That also induces breathing. Another thing is the arm movements, which suggest those of swimming. Manipulate the patient's arms in that manner while he is lying on his face. This also helps the chest to expand and contract. A cold dash of water over the face is stimulating. When you think there is a slight sign of consciousness, commence saying, "Breathe deeper, take more air into your lungs." And the likelihood is that he will do so.

Q. What is the cause of fainting?

A. Fainting may have various immediate causes, such as over-exertion, strong emotion, stomach dilation. Fainting, fundamentally, is caused by an anaemic condition of the brain, a sudden want of blood in the neural centers. Therefore, anyone who feels dizzy or about to swoon should at once hang the head down and hold the breath for a minute. Get the head lower than the body, and take long, deep breaths. In order to have a permanent and complete cure, you must live on natural foods.

Q. I get fainting spells during the day. I have at one time drunk a great deal of tea. Could this be the cause of my weakness?

A. Tannin (tannic acid) in the system acts like uric acid, and the possibility is that there is some connection between fainting and tea drinking. When you feel faintness coming on, go out into the cool air and commence deep breathing. Or go into the bathroom and take a cold shower. After you have wet yourself once over, get out and rub yourself down with a towel; then get under the shower again. Do that three or four times and your whole system will be stimulated into activity and the fainting spell will be warded off.

FASTING

Q. Do you approve of fasting to clean the system?

A. Fasting is a very important subject, for I find that most people fast wrongly. They do not know how to begin or when to stop, nor do they know why they fast. To begin with, fasting will give your digestive system a rest, and you may depend upon it that whenever the digestive organs complain, they need a rest. Now, if you let them take a one-day rest, you will get really hungry. Hunger is one of the best tonics ever invented. If there is then any undigested food still in your system, it will certainly be absorbed in short order. Fasting means abstaining from food, and that, in turn, means hunger, which is your tonic. Your digesive organs, once rested, commence to call for food. That call is termed "hunger."

But when you ignore this desire and do not satisfy the craving of your digestive tract, these organs commence to relax; this continuous demand for food will stop; that is, your hunger will disappear. Then you are merely hibernating, and there is no benefit at all in that —quite the contrary. Say you fast for one day. This is safe enough. Then, if you continue for a second and a third day, your hunger will mount up. But if you abstain from eating anything at all at the end of the three-day period, your hunger will leave you at that point. If you continue the fast further, there is no tonic effect; there is even a real danger involved. The bowels, not having in them a filler to keep them dilated, are liable to friction and irritation. This irritation by peristaltic action will cause a fever, and perhaps the casting off of a great deal of the inflamed membrane. Nothing to be especially alarmed about here, but if this goes on until it causes the outer fibre of the nerve tissues to break down with it, then, I say, beware, you are doing something injurious. I do not consider long-continued fasting safe. There should be no continuous fasting after five days' abstinence, and I do not advise total fasting under any circumstances. Take liquids—water or fruit juices—on the day that you do not take solids. If anyone desires to fast, this is the most rational and safest way.

A fast is a splendid thing for the digestive organs. Sometimes we are compelled to put people on a fast for diseases of the stomach or bowels. You cannot get the stomach well unless you let it rest. Nevertheless, you must give it the wherewithal at the same time to cure the ulcer or other affliction. Food, nothing else, will do the trick. Healing can take place only with proper foods. Fast, therefore, one day on liquids. When you feel hunger coming on, take a drink. That will still it for a while. It will come again; then take another drink. A good idea is to take a glassful of either water or fruit juice every two hours, but absolutely no tea, coffee, chocolate, milk, or buttermilk. These are fermentable and gas forming. Besides, you have no thymus gland with which to digest milk.

When you fast on liquids, your schedule should be as follows: fruit juices or water until noon; vegetable juices or water the rest of the day. Vegetable juices include pineapple juice and rhubarb juice. These liquids are all nourishing but not filling. They will stir up your hunger; in fact, you will be as hungry as a bear. The next day you eat. Choose your fruit. Eat what you want. Drink between meals such liquids as you like best, but only up to half an hour before meals or when two hours have elapsed after meals. Liquids will interfere with proper digestion of food.

If you would like to try a more stringent fast, take

liquids for two days, and, on the third day, solids, for two weeks. Your hunger will be much keener. You will feel as though you could not wait for the first dish, but that is a good thing, as I said before. When you then eat solid foods, they will act as a brush, will sweep out the digestive tract. Moreover, the digestive organs will have rested, so that they will get all the nourishment out of the food you eat.

For a still more stringent fast, try three days of liquids and one of solids, for three weeks. You can get along on four days of liquids and one of solids, or on five days of liquids and one day solids, for four or five weeks, if you want to, but from patients' reports, the most favorable way is two days liquids and one day solids, or three days liquids and one day solids. Some get the best results with two days and others with three, but very few go beyond that.

After you have had one day of liquids and one day of solids for a week or two and you still want to continue fasting, try two days on liquids and one day on solids, for two weeks. When those two weeks are up, you might, if still dissatisfied with results, try three days of liquids and one of solids, for another week. You will find this general method more satisfactory than straight fasting. If you do as I have suggested, you will create hunger. When you are four or five days along on a conventional fast, you have no more desire for food. What is it that creates hunger? Eating. So eat every other day, or every third, fourth, or fifth day, if you want to, but there should be no wider spread than that, for then you would consume your own flesh, and this can do much harm.

Q. After eating nothing but fruits and vegetables, uncooked for some time, nothing tastes good to me. Would you advise me to go back to my old diet?

A. No, I would simply let myself go hungry for a little while; I would let myself starve for a bit. Then I would find out if my digestive organs would not like some fruit—and I think they would. There is nothing that we cannot learn to eat when we are hungry, and enjoy it. Just put hunger into your system and you will think that raw foods are the best you have ever eaten in your life. Once you acquire the live food habit, you will not get tired of it. Everything is always wholesome and fresh. There is, of course, a saturation point, but it will not take long for you to get your taste back.

Q. Is it necessary to take enemas while fasting?

A. With my method of fasting, you do not need enemas, because food days alternate with fast days. In this manner, the bowels remain in good condition and do not require artificial stimulation or mechanical action.

Q. I have been on an orange juice fast for three days. What would you advise me to break my fast on?

A. That depends upon the time of day. If you break your fast in the morning, start with fruit; if you do it at noon, then eat a lettuce leaf or two; and if you break your fast in the evening, try grated carrots. In the morning, start, say, with only one orange. Wait an hour or so, and if you feel no distress, eat two more. Then wait another hour, and if nothing disagreeable happens, you may satisfy your hunger fully as regards oranges. At noon, eat lettuce, first a little and then increasing quantities as your stomach seems to demand.

Speaking generally, it is better to eat bulky foods like lettuce, rather than oranges, which contain a great deal of liquid, and for that reason furnish less material for bowel dilation. Not only that, but lettuce and all the herbs and roots are tissue builders to a greater extent than the fruits, and hence are of great value when you are beginning to rebuild your body.

Q. Is the alternate-day fasting system the best and quickest way to cure all diseases?

A. You cannot cure starvation diseases by fasting. Most diseases are caused by eating foodless foods. If you wish to get well, start eating Nature's foods, unprocessed, chock full of life. Heavy elimination is often reduced by fasting, when desired. Generally speaking, eating is more pleasant as well as more profitable, within limits.

FEET AND ANKLES

Q. What causes ankles to swell?

A. Kidney trouble, likely. It means that there is an excess of water in the blood as the kidneys are not in working order. If, when you press your finger into the swelling and pull it out again, the hole remains there for some time, it means your kidneys are not working properly. They need washing out with the kind of food that will do the work. Both cucumbers and tomatoes are splendid remedies for weak, diseased kidneys. Asparagus and raw peanuts, too, are excellent; also melons of various kinds.

However, in some instances, rheumatism is the cause of the trouble. If such be the case, take Epsom salt baths and eat natural foods exclusively. Regardless of whether the cause be kidney trouble or rheumatism, your case demands plenty of air, water, sun baths, and stimulation of the blood circulation by massage. You soon will notice considerable improvement.

Q. How should I treat my ankles? They have been swollen since I sprained them some years ago.

A. Your blood must be a very poor healing agent if your sprain is still in evidence. It is high time you commenced to live on natural food. It is true that there are people who are still suffering from injuries incurred as long as twelve years ago. Why? Because there is no healing substance in their blood. Their blood is so bad it can just barely keep them on their feet, without being able to do any repairing. In such cases you must be very careful to eat only foods that offer real building material to the blood.

Q. Is there a remedy for fallen arches aside from exercises?

A. The exercises will do you a great deal of good provided your diet is right. The treatment I recommend for fallen arches is to soak your feet for twenty minutes or half an hour in hot water, just as hot as you can endure. After your feet have been in long enough to become red with blood, dip them into cold water for a minute, wipe dry, and walk on tiptoe until you get tired. A good thing to do is to walk upstairs on tiptoe, then down again, backwards. Do this until you become tired; then go to bed. Do it every night. You will soon get strong insteps. Your foot muscles are weak. That means you must live on such food as will help to strengthen them. Also rub your feet with olive oil occasionally.

Many more people are flat-footed than we often imagine. This trouble is caused by the sinking down of the tarsal bones, small narrow bones between the middle and outside toes, the cause of their giving away being weakness of the tendons and muscles that cannot hold these bones in their proper position. All of this is derived from eating foods that have in them little or no organic salts, which are necessary to keep our human skeleton in proper condition. They are found only in uncooked roots, fruits, and herbs.

Methods of support, such as insoles, or metal devices, have been contrived to raise the broken-down arch up to its normal position. Temporary relief is given the sufferer, but never the restored arch he really wants. On the contrary, as long as cooked food is eaten, the muscles and ligaments will remain weak. Cooked mineral salts are always dead and cannot therefore be built up into strong muscular tissue. Live food, on the other hand, does produce strong muscles and tissue, especially the root vegetables.

To restore a natural arch, live on live foods for at least six months in order to correct your blood. A pure bloodstream is always fundamentally necessary to the building of a strong body and a sound mind. If your blood is good, your arteries, veins, lungs, heart, and all other organs, will possess dynamic power and aid your muscles to frame the outside of your body in a pleasing and efficient way.

Q. What is the cause and remedy for sweating feet?

A. Most people eat too much salt, which in turn makes them drink too much water. This water has to be expelled somehow, and the feet are convenient for the purpose, especially if you wear leather or rubber shoes, shutting out the air as they do. Ventilate your feet. Why not go barefooted? Seriously speaking, it is a waste of money to buy shoes. We do not need them. They cripple our feet, create unwholesome smells, and shut out life-giving air. Some men and women have courage enough to wear sandals, or no shoes at all, and this is exceedingly sensible. Certainly, you may go about at home minus shoes. Also, sun your feet every day, if you can.

Q. What is good for sore feet?

A. See that your shoes are right. When you buy a pair of shoes, have plenty of toe room. Your feet should be fan-shaped, broad side front, not twisted to one side. For soreness, take a hot foot bath for half an hour, as hot as possible. When you get through, thrust the feet into cold water. Rub dry, and go to bed.

Q. Do you know of a sure cure for soft and hard corns?

A. Did you ever think that if you wore no shoes you would not have any corns? You are so accus-tomed to wearing shoes that you do not think this has anything to do with it. If you must have them, adjust your shoes to the foot, not the foot to the shoes. Be sure you get shoes that bind only in the instep, that give your toes and ankle plenty of room. The shoe should also have plenty of ventilation. You really ought to go barefooted as much as you reasonably can. As for the corns, put some lemon juice on them, or a little kerosene oil after you have soaked them in hot water. Do this every night, and soon you will not have corns any longer. However, if you do not have shoes that fit you, new corns will soon appear. The same treatment applies for callous spots as well. Do not cut, but soak off.

Q. Can my broken-down meditarsal arch be attributed to my excess weight—nearly 200 pounds; normal, 130?

A. You should go a step beyond that and ask: "Can my excess weight be attributed to wrong living?" Then I would answer "Yes" to both questions.

Q. Would you advise women to wear heels as flat as men's? They do not look graceful to me.

A. There may be cases of girl babies being born with naturally higher heels than male children. If so, they have escaped my attention. I do not believe that our Mother Nature has destined women, even in a shoeless world, to be less graceful and agile than men. Doubtless the Chinese foot-binders also had designs for improving upon natural workmanship. Their ideas, however, of late, have gone the way that ours, relative to high heels, will go with the development of real intelligence.

Q. My ankles and feet have rough, whitish skin, rather chronic. What would you advise?

A. Very likely this is excess elimination. Bathe in cold water; use mud baths and olive oil rubs.

FERMENTATION

Q. Do natural foods ferment?

A. A ferment is the deoxidization and disorganization of any carbohydrate. Cooked carbohydrates of all kinds inevitably cause ferments when eaten. As to flesh food, gangrene sets in twenty minutes after the animal is killed. That is the beginning of ferment in meat carbohydrates. Fermentation can be held up somewhat by soaking the flesh in alum water. The simplest way is to soak in alcohol or any stable solution. Salt water will do. The salt is as stable as rock. It cannot digest.

There are two kinds of ferment—sweet and sour. The sour is dangerous and destructive. The sweet is harmless, though annoying. What can we do to stop ferment? All the herbs, like lettuce, celery, spinach, watercress, cabbage, dandelion, are non-fermentable. Onions and garlic, however, produce a sweet ferment, not a sour one. Roots do not ferment—that is, all those which do not belong to the onion family. Beets, carrots, potatoes, parsnips, turnips, radishes, all are non-fermentable and very rich in earth salts. Many of you may have eaten non-fermentable herbs or roots and immediately afterward suffered from gas. Why? It has not come from the food. No, you have stored up phlegm in the digestive tract which the digestion of the food in the stomach breaks up, and it is this phlegm, worked into ether, that is causing fermentation. The digestive organs, with their peristaltic movements, churn this leafy or root food you have eaten, and the contents of the stomach breaks up the phlegmy coating everywhere about, causing ferment. This ether evaporates, and some of it discharges. This is annoying, but get rid of bad rubbish. Keep right on, and you will soon be through with all this. There is no ferment in your food.

Many a person beginning with my instructions, comes to me in a few days and says: "Doctor, I seem to be getting worse instead of better." Excellent! The stomach is getting rid of a catarrhal condition. Continue, for you are house-cleaning. When you are clean and pure, there will be power of absorption and assimilation. The villi of the digestive tract have been covered up and paralyzed. When they are uncovered, they will begin to perform their functions; namely, the absorption and assimilation of food. When you once have this phlegm cleaned out, you will have won a great victory, for then your body can commence to assimilate natural live food and create good blood. That is one of the greatest possible victories toward health.

Q. Milk ferments and tomatoes ferment. Will you please explain the difference?

A. Cooking a tomato fixes the acid. Then it will

ferment. But a raw tomato will not ferment unless taken in too large quantities. All fruits and herbal fruits (the tomato belongs in this latter classification) will ferment if you overload your stomach, however delicious they may be. Why not eat just enough? Then you will never suffer. Hunger is the test. If you are not hungry, your stomach can not use any more food. Milk, unlike the tomato, causes a sour ferment, which is dangerous.

FEVER

Q. I have for five months had a high temperature, from 100° to 130°, pulse 115° in the afternoon, together with low vitality. What shall I do?

A. In this case, take only liquids. Never eat solids when you have a fever. You may drink as much liquid as you care for, fruit and vegetable juices diluted one-half with water. Remember, take your fruit juices from morning until noon, vegetable juices from noon until evening, and nothing at all when you have a very high temperature.

Practice deep breathing, too. Breathe in slowly and deeply. When you have an opportunity, take sun baths for half an hour or one hour between nine and twelve in the morning, minus all clothes.

Q. What causes excessive perspiration accompanied by enervation?

A. You are undergoing eliminative fever in which the body is burning up waste matter. Excessive perspiration spells weakness. It should be stopped, or you will become exhausted. For this, take alternate warm and cold baths. Fill a tub with blood-warm water, and have a bowl with cold water near it. Bathe in the warm water; then get out and sponge off with cold water. Afterward, go back into the warm. Alternate in this way for half an hour.

Q. What is the cause of dry lips?

A. Fever.

Q. Why do I develop a fever when I stop eating, as in a fast?

A. Because waste matter in you is burning up. Get rid of the waste matter and you will have no fever. If much of the waste matter is coming out through your skin, take an Epsom salt bath once a week.

Q. What foods are advised in cases of ordinary fever?

A. Currant juice is especially good for fever. Be sure, if you use the dried variety, that they are unsulphured. Do not eat any solids whatever.

Q. Is ague a curable disease?

A. Ague is a malarial fever, with alternate hot and cold spells. This is one of the easiest of all diseases to cure, and yet many doctors say it has to run its course. To run its course means that if the patient has great vitality, he will probably win out in from one to three weeks, but if he has little vitality, he is apt to drag along for two or three months, and finish up in a pitiably weak condition. Nature's method gets him well in from two to three days. The patient should not touch any solids for three days, having liquids and fruit juices only. After three days he may eat something tender and delicious, like lettuce, to break the fast.

If you live on natural foods, you will never get ague. I do not care if you live in steaming swamps, you cannot contract it if you will do this. It is indeed worth while to know for yourself the real value of natural foods, foods that were given us from the very beginning of human life, the sunshine kindling them, being stored, as it were, in semi-permanent form for our use.

FOOD COMBINATIONS

Q. What do you mean by "blending" a salad?

A. Drink a glass of lemonade, then a glass of milk, and you will certainly have a stomach ache. That is because blending is trying to take place in the stomach. Some kind of harmony will come, finally, but it is going to kick up a fuss first. That is colic. However, take the same lemonade and milk, pour them together in the air, let them blend before drinking, and they will not hurt you. I do not recommend milk, however, because it is a ferment and a natural culture for all forms of aerial bacteria and bacilli.

Liquids blend almost instantly. With other foods, such as lettuce and tomatoes, blending goes on slowly. You must blend these, because tomatoes are a fruit and lettuce is a vegetable. Of course, you can eat them together at once, but you will not feel just right afterwards. Cube the tomatoes, chop the lettuce medium fine, mix well, and let stand for an hour. That is a blended salad. The air is a wonderful adjuster, and if you can get some sunshine onto the food, that will be another great aid. Set the food in the sunshine when mixed. If mixtures are cut medium fine, they will blend faster than if coarse. Though a sick person should never have a mixture of fruit and vegetables, usually he has been so perverted in his tastes by the use of cooked foods that you must imitate some of these through complex mixtures before he will feel at home with the new diet.

Time is required to blend some things, for instance, fruits, nuts, and vegetables mixed together. They will have to blend two hours or more. For example, beets are quite hard even when ground, and it requires a long time for the rhubarb juice to soak through the fibre. It would be well to grind up the beet at night, cover it with rhubarb juice, and let soak all night. After you have done that, you have something that is very delicious.

Q. May all live foods be combined?

A. Be more careful when mixing live foods than cooked foods, because it makes no difference how you mix cooked foods, since they are inactive substances anyway, but natural foods have living properties. Fruits and nuts both grow on trees, and hence are congenial, but do not mix nuts and fruits with vegetables, unless you let them blend. Even in such a case, remember you are only tickling your palate. Try not to mix foods at all. Eat one thing at a time, in its natural state, for each kind of food is a perfect combination in itself. The one most pleasing to your taste is the one that has the right mixture for you at the time, and is composed of the elements that you need to get and stay well. It is in harmony with all the vibrations of the earth, particularly that of the locality in which it grew. If it grew in New York, then it is food for you when you are in New York. If you go to Panama, eat the fruits and vegetables that grow there. You will then be immune to climatic fevers.

Q. Is it all right to eat honey with tomatoes? If not, what would be advisable?

A. Yes, honey may be eaten with any kind of food. Honey and oil are two things that may be eaten with any fruit, vegetable, or nut.

Q. Will strawberries combine with fruit?

A. Yes, with fruits, but not with vegetables. Strawberries and flaked nuts will also go well together, but never mix cereals or vegetables with fruits, unless you let them blend before eating.

Q. Does green sweet corn mix with carob and tomatoes?

A. I would rather mix my corn with carrots, turnips, and parsnips, but carob and tomatoes go very nicely. Sweet corn is a cereal and carob a leguminous fruit. The best mixture, however, is no mixture at all!

Q. What should one blend with fresh sweet corn to make it palatable?

A. You do not need anything to make fresh sweet

corn palatable. However, there is some difference in varieties of corn. A good dressing for corn is a kind of lemon cheese. To a tablespoonful of raw peanut butter, add lemon juice. Work it in until it gets cheese-like and white as snow. Put that on your corn and it will be very delicious.

Q. How does pineapple compare in value with other vegetables?

A. It makes a delicious dressing and a wonderful food when chipped with cabbage, or lettuce, or other vegetable combination, but be sure you get fresh, not canned, pineapple.

Q. What combines well with your wholewheat and olive bread?

A. Wholewheat bread may be eaten with our pemi-ken or any other cereal, including corn, but do not eat it with vegetables or fruit.

Q. Are bananas good with strawberries?

A. That is a splendid combination: both are fruits.

Q. I have heard about soaking dried fruits in water before using. Is that advisable?

A. Dried fruits should never be eaten in a dried condition. They should always be soaked in water and re-freshened before eating, for their sugars are too concentrated for the best results. You should dilute their sugar to its original state. A dried fig is sweeter than a fig taken directly from the tree. Estimate the amount of water that has evaporated from it (some

80 or 90 per cent of its weight), add this to your figs, and let it soak into your fruit. After three or four hours, eat it. So with raisins—soak them in water before using.

Q. Do coconut and raw pumpkin combine well?

A. Coconut is a fruit, and grows on a tree. The pumpkin is also a fruit, but grows on a ground vine. Fruit always combines with fruit, and if you think that coconut goes well with pumpkin, eat it. Pumpkin is very wholesome, one of the best foods for curing tuberculosis.

Q. Can you suggest some good fruit combinations?

A. Cut oranges into small pieces, sprinkle over some almonds, add a little honey, and eat. Cut an avocado into little square sections. Mix with an equal amount of rosy tomatoes. You will not need anything else in addition to either of these combinations for a balanced meal.

Q. Do you advise eating starch and protein to-gether?

A. How are you going to separate starch from pro-tein? All starchy foods contain protein, and all pro-tein foods contain starch. Peanuts contain protein, and the finest quality of starch as well.

Q. Why should we not eat fruits with vegetables?

A. Because fruits ferment when combined with vegetables. Vibration theories tell us that the fruit is electric and vegetables magnetic. This causes constant interaction until fully blended, either outside of, or in, the stomach.

Q. Does rhubarb juice mix well with raw sweet potatoes?

A. Yes, rhubarb is a vegetable, and so are potatoes and sweet potatoes. You may mix them very nicely. Rhubarb juice makes a fine dressing for vegetables of all kinds. Lemon juice, being a fruit extract, is best used on fruits, like the avocado.

FOOD—COOKED

Q. When one suffers from asthma of long standing and has practically lived on natural food without getting relief, what else can be done?

A. It may be that you are eating a breakfast of live food, but dinner and supper cooked. What are you really doing? The cooked food ferments because it is acid. Everything cooked is fixed in its nature and is not soluble. It does not digest by absorption and assimilation, but, for the most part, decays. The result of this fermentation is powerful acid, and when you take natural raw foods the next morning, the acid in the stomach clashes with the acid in the fruit. What good does that do? You may as well cook all three meals. You are going up a ladder for one meal and going down the ladder at the next meal, up again and down. How, then, can you advance? You must progress, not stand still. If one meal of live food will do you good, why not eat all of them uncooked?

Q. Will such foods as rice, wheat, spinach, etc.,

cooked in a tightly covered can at a temperature of 185° to 195°, lose any of their nutritive value?

A. If you want live food, you must not box it up and cook it. You may cook it in earthen jars, glass, enamel, porcelain, whatever you please, but the life is going to come out. It is a form of magnetism, and will penetrate a sheet of glass ten feet wide. Anything that is able to penetrate that glass will penetrate steel or any other metal. You cannot house up life.

FRUIT AND VEGETABLE CULTURE

Q. What causes fruit flies and vegetable pests?

A. I was once bothered with parasites in my garden, but no more, since I have the soil thoroughly cleansed. Parasites are caused by the wrong kind of fertilizer. If California would use decomposed finely-ground granite for fertilizer, instead of barnyard manure, it would do away with flies and pests of all kinds.

Q. What is the best fertilizer to use for gardens and orchards?

A. Fresh manure from animals should never be used, for it is not sufficiently decomposed. It must be two or three years old, or even older in some cases. The food raised on ground so fertilized will be normal and unharrassed by parasites. What the insects really do is to clean house after raw fertilizer has been used. They breed in the manure and help in its decomposition.

Q. What do you consider the most natural work for man?

A. One of the most ancient books of record in the world, the Hebrew Bible, speaks of paradise as a garden, the only work of its inhabitants being the trimming and general culture of the trees. This conception of the earliest work of mankind is shared by other primitive records, such as the Buddhist and ancient religious writings of India. These days of prehistoric innocence are looked upon universally as representing the ideal occupation of mankind. The Golden Age is life in a garden or orchard.

So much for legend. From the modern scientific standpoint, man should work in the out-of-doors, not at monotonous drudgery, but in genial cooperation with Nature in her most beneficent aspects. In fruit culture, for instance, the struggle with weeds is minimized. There are no chemical fumes or physical hazards involved when natural methods of horticulture are used, the nerves are relaxed, power of digestion strengthened, and the air is full of oxygen instead of exhaust gas. Large-scale methods of cultivation are not excluded. On the contrary, we believe in cooperative enterprise involving the use of labor-saving machinery. Who, visualizing the future America as one vast orchard and garden, would not concede that this were an improvement over the America of today, with its denuded forests, abandoned farms, and vacant lots, from the standpoint of beauty as well as utility?

FRUITS AND FRUIT DIET

Q. Can man live on fruits alone?

A. I am going to give you my candid opinion. A

beginner on natural foods who tries at once to live on fruits, is likely to go insane before long. Let him, rather, start on fruits in the morning, herbs at noon, and roots at night, and live in that way until his body is rebuilt. Thoroughly strengthened with the strong tissue cells derived from vegetables, fruits, and nuts, he will then be completely rebuilt. Man's mental and physical equipment has been so perverted by cooked-food eating that should he put it under a too sudden and severe strain, he would become mentally unbalanced, handicapped by a weak body as he is. First build a one hundred per cent body. Then you may try the radical fruitarian diet if you wish.

Fruits alone have too little material for tissue building. Vegetables and roots contain these in abundance. Fruits are a wonderful food, but only for people who are perfectly clean, who have never been polluted by wrong eating; people who have never known anything about disease, being naturally normal and healthy, full of vigor and pep; people who are immune from any disease.

Q. Is there any fruit that is a body builder?

A. Yes, all fruits are body builders; they build and maintain, but are not as strong and powerful in that respect as vegetables. Vegetables are the best builders because they get the richest earth salts directly from the soil. Potatoes, parsnips, turnips, beets, carrots, and the radish, all have their edible portion hidden in the soil. When they are in the ground, they are in darkness. The body makes repairs when you are asleep, also during hours of darkness When you are asleep, your

subconscious mind takes the food that you get in dark·
ness and from darkness to do the necessary repair work.
Is not that harmony? Eat your fruit in the morning to
fully awaken you — oranges, possibly, one or a half
dozen. They grow on trees, far from the ground. At
noon eat your lettuce, or other herbs, also daylight
food, but growing close to the ground. They are better
builders and are magnetic as well. At night, three or
four hours before bedtime, eat your roots. These are
formed directly in the ground. They contain pure
starch, but it is raw, and hence always good.

Q. Are bananas wholesome?

A. Many a physician has said that bananas are indigestible. They are so when they are green, but the
same banana, when ripe, is very nourishing. It should
have black spots all over it. The best way to test for
ripeness is to look at the tip. Sometimes you find a
speckled skin but a green tip. Do not eat these, but
wait until all is yellow; then they are fit for food. Buy
your bananas on the stalk, if you possibly can (as large
a section as you require), and let them ripen in your
home. You will be surprised at the sweet flavor and
the thinness of the peel.

Q. Are bananas mucous-forming food? In case of
colitis, is it advisable to take two bananas daily, mashed
and diluted with water?

A. Colitis is an inflammation of the colon. You then
want something that is very soft and tender, and the
sugar and starch of the banana are not harmful to the
inflamed tissues, but will help the cure along. Be sure

that your bananas are ripe, the skins well speckled.

Q. Why do bananas cause a temperature every time I eat them? I eat them with almonds and honey.

A. They contain much starch and sugar, and with honey make a splendid warming food. If you get a bit too warm after eating, it must be due to some congestion in the digestive tract, some ferment to be gotten rid of by burning.

Q. I like tomatoes very much. Please advise me when and how to eat them.

A. The tomato is a fruit, rich in organic salts, with a fine, stimulating acid when not cooked. Remember that no acid fruits must ever be cooked, for cooking fixes the acidity. These fixed acids invariably cause acidosis, and many times, as a result, sudden death. Best of all, eat tomatoes alone, and for your breakfast, since they are a fruit. If you desire, however, you may mince them and use as a dressing on lettuce, spinach, or other leafy vegetable, but you will have to let this mixture blend for from half an hour to an hour, according to the toughness of the vegetable fiber with which you mix them. You may also eat them in combination with other fruits, according to taste.

Q. Are tomatoes and watermelon vegetables or fruits?

A. Tomatoes are a fruit, not a vegetable. The pineapple, on the other hand, is a vegetable, not a fruit. The tomato is the fruit of a vinal herb; so are the watermelon, pumpkin, squash, and cucumber. The most nourishing of all fruit. is the tomato; next in order is the cucumber. Cucumbers and tomatoes, by the way, make a splendid comLination.

Q. Is the persimmon a fruit or a vegetable?

A. It is a tree fruit, one of the tastiest. There is no fruit so delightfully rich, delicious, and perfect, as the persimmon. They were once considered a sacred fruit. Then, too, they are very easily digested. The persimmon tree in fall, when its fruit is ripe, is a fine spectacle.

Q. Is watermelon a good food?

A. If you like watermelon, eat all you want, but with it you need some basic food. Flake some nuts and mix with honey. Eat about three ounces of this as a side dish to your melon. The green near the rind is valuable for its mineral salts. Eat a little of it. It is a tissue builder, containing organic sodium chloride, and in the center of the melon is real grape sugar. Eat watermelon seeds and all, but do not chew the seeds; swallow them whole. The seed is rich in silicon, a lubricant for the joints and for the synovial membrane. The silicon you want is on the surface of the seed. Joints, when well lubricated, will not crack when you knee bend, nor will they grind. As there are no sharp corners on these seeds, they will drive down through the intestines, acting as roughage. You will find it very beneficial to thus clean out the twenty-five feet of small intestines and five feet of colon. Such a breakfast of watermelon and flaked nuts with honey, will keep you satisfied all morning. If you ate no nuts, you would probably be hungry again in two hours.

Q. What is the food value of the fig?

A. Figs are cultivated in all semi-tropical and tropical countries, and are very nutritious. They are rich in grape sugar, a laxative. Californians have produced what is called the Kadota fig, which contains only about one-third or half as much seed as ordinary figs. It is sweeter, and more juicy, and has a richer flavor than the common variety. Though I have said it is a laxative, do not think that such purging is inevitable. I find that with some people prunes have a very good effect on the bowels, while others will get better results from the fig. Prunes, in general, are not considered as laxative in effect as the fig, but it is evident that in some cases prunes are really more so. Every individual is to some extent a law unto himself. Your master builders, the tastebuds, always select correctly the food you should eat. Do not ask anyone what is good for this and that, but ask yourself, "What natural food do I crave most?"

Q. Does fruit create acids in the stomach?

A. No. You may eat oranges, grapefruit, pears, lemons, or any other fruit, with impunity; not one of them will produce an acid reaction. The lemon, for instance, the strongest acid fruit that grows, when perfectly ripe, may be rolled and eaten "as is." It will turn into sugar in a few seconds. Lemon exposed to the air is acid, but just put it into your mouth and notice how quickly it will taste like sugar.

There is a great difference between cooked and live food acids. If you should cook that acid lemon and then eat it, it would blister your throat and stomach, and would in fact be dangerous. The cooked tomato, for its part, is saturated with citric acid, and therefore is really a mild poison, not a food. Tomato acid, when cooked, destroys the red corpuscles, thus paving the way for anaemia.

Q. Should a person with thin blood abstain from eating citrus fruit?

A. Citrus fruits do thin the blood, to advantage when the warmer season is here. In the winter, we have fruits that are much better for retaining body heat. They are: apples, dried figs, dates, and prunes, as well as avocados, nuts, and bananas.

Q. Is the peel of citrus fruits edible?

A. Nature has provided this peel with acid and turpentine to protect the interior from insects. If you squeeze lemon or orange peel and apply a match, there will be a tiny explosion caused by the turpentine mixed with ethereal nitre. The insects do not like the acrid taste, and will leave the fruit severely alone. The peel, with some people, has a laxative effect.

Q. Will you please tell us about the food value of the avocado?

A. Of all fruits, the avocado is the most valuable. The avocado is a brain food in the true sense of the word. It aids the memory, makes you a keen thinker, and nourishes all nerve tissues of the brain. It is, oddly enough, also the finest remedy for female weakness, or male prostate trouble. Avocados contain only two per cent protein, but an abundance of fat. They contain plenty of chlorophyll, and chlorophyll is a splendid protein. They contain much phosphorous, which is the element used particularly by the brain.

Q. Why is it that apples do not agree with me, while other fruits and vegetables produce no bad effect?

A. If you like the taste of apples, even though they cause you trouble, eat more apples. If you like them, they have something for you. If a whole one distresses you, take only one half, or one quarter. Keep on until you can eat a whole apple, and more.

Q. Is the carob bean a good food for humans?

A. The carob bean (St. John's bread) is a leguminous fruit, 50 per cent sugar and 14 per cent protein. It is very rich in silicon, roughage, and cellulose, which makes it a very good muscle builder, good for constipation—really a complete food.

If you can eat the whole carob bean, do so, but if you cannot, have it made into a meal. People once had strong teeth and could eat carob beans, but now that is impossible for many. You can make confections out of carob by mixing with dried fruit, or you may make a drink out of it, or uncooked bread. It has a delicious flavor.

Q. What is the best time of day to eat coconut, and should it be eaten with fruits and vegetables?

A. Morning is the best time, or you may eat it at

noon. Eat with fruits, for it is a real nut. Nearly any fruit will go nicely with coconut, but the best way to eat it is alone, as with other foods.

Q. What good or harm is there in eating cactus pears?

A. There is an edible cactus pear which is very tasty; also cactus candy, which in most cases, however, has been spoiled by cooking. The Mexicans use also the plant itself, removing the spiny exterior, and cutting into cubes for use in salads.

Q. Will you tell me how lemons can be kept fresh in a dry climate?

A. The best way to keep your lemons is to put them into a keg filled with water. Every two or three days, empty and fill with fresh water.

Q. Are skins of fruits and vegetables good to eat?

A. Often the most nutritious elements lie nearest or in the skin, as in apples, pears, potatoes, carrots. Besides, the skin, passing through the colon, serves as splendid roughage. If you have reason to suspect that there is any spray material on the fruit or vegetable, wash it carefully before eating. However, the danger of spray poison has been much exaggerated. As for germs on the peel, the alkalis and acids of the digestive tract will take care of these very nicely.

FRUITS—DRIED

Q. I have a chance to get some olives off a tree. Please tell me how I can dry and prepare them.

A. Lay them on a cloth, or on screens, in the sun;

turn them over now and then. Dry them to the point where when put into the mouth and bitten, they will break. Then they are dry enough. The best way to pick them is to put a canvas around the tree and shake them down. Pick them about the first of January. Some varieties may be ripe in December, but as a rule we seldom think of getting any oil from olives until February or March.

Q. Is there more energy in green vegetables than in nuts and dried fruits? If so, why?

A. There is more energy in fresh fruits and vegetables than in the dried or preserved form of that particular fruit or vegetable. Dry your fruit and you are concentrating a certain element in it, and at the same time you waste something that you need. You never can get back that same water you have taken out of the fruits when you dried them. You can add other water, but it is never the same. Steaming, vaporizing, drying —all this can do no good. Get your vegetables directly from the garden and your fruits from the grove. That is the best and most wholesome food. Some dried fruits can be restored to a tasty condition by soaking them, and vegetables likewise, but they are never the same. The coconut is our only fresh nut. All nuts are energy-builders, but they should be eaten sparingly, and always flaked.

Q. Can one preserve tomatoes by drying them, and how is it done?

A. Yes. Slice them, but not too thin. Slice a me dium-sized tomato about three times, leaving the mid dle slice a little thicker than the ends. Lay on a waxed paper so as not to lose too much moisture, and handle them very gently. Dried tomatoes are very tasty, but if you can get fresh tomatoes all year 'round, as we can here in Southern California, eat them.

Q. Are the figs, dates, and prunes on sale at health food stores, processed?

A. Prunes are run through hot lye water to quicken the drying process. They are practically cooked. Passing one of these processing plants in harvest season, you will be greeted by the odor of cooking prunes, reminiscent of your own kitchen range while you still had one.

Figs are sometimes steamed, and the light varieties, such as the Calimyrna and Kadota, are occasionally sulphured to give them a uniform light color, although the pure food law requires such sulphuring to be indicated upon the package. Oftentimes, however, they are sold in bulk, and it is up to the purchaser to make certain of what he is buying. Fumigation is required by state law.

As for dates, they are usually processed, either by the use of sulphur fumes or powdered sulphur. Get, if you can, the celophane-packaged "fresh" dates, direct from the tree. These should be available all over the United States and Canada in the fall and early winter. They melt in the mouth and are truly delicious, a natural confection. Such dates are usually not processed at all.

Should dried fruits, then, be eaten? The answer is: not if the fresh fruit is available. However, such dried fruit, unsulphured, of course, is a fairly natural product and may form a legitimate part of the live-fooder's dietary when used in moderate quantities. The high sugar content will make such food valuable, especially in colder climates, and generally during the cooler season. Soak before eating until the approximate amount of evaporated moisture is replaced. Never use sulphured dried fruit. The fruit has a lighter color, but sulphur has an extremely irritating effect upon the digestive tract and eliminative organs. When your tastebuds are once educated, you will be able to detect the use of sulphur dioxide by a distinct "flatness" or "deadness" of flavor.

Q. What fruits may be dried successfully? Do you recommend drying, rather than canning?

A. After fresh fruits, nothing is more delicious and healthful than dried apples, peaches, pears, prunes, apricots, nectarines, cherries, and so on down the list. If you have a surplus of fresh fruit and wish a first-rate menu throughout the winter, a little labor, plus sunlight, will perform wonders. You can get labor-saving devices, such as slicers and pit extractors, very reasonably these days. Canning destroys the life, whereas drying retains it, in addition to storing up, as it were, sunshine. In the process of canning, even in so-called cold-packs, heating is required by steam or hot water.

GALL BLADDER

Q. How can one get rid of gall stones?

A. Remove the cause, which is salt-eating—all varieties, not merely table salt. If you are eating biscuits which contain baking soda (saleratus, bicarbonate of soda), you are paving the way for hardening of the arteries, gall stones, and sclerosis of the liver. Do not brush your teeth with tooth powder, for thereby more salt goes into your stomach. Get your salt organically, as it grows in spinach or cabbage. Get it in its natural form as living salt.

Q. Will you please answer my question? I have a pain under my right shoulder blade, and a tender spot between the navel and rib. If it is gall stones or gall bladder trouble, how can I cure it?

A. If you have gall stones, you will have intense pain. The gall bladder will discharge stones at times, causing much distress. Take one-half cup of pure olive oil, and with a very hot cloth absorb some and place over the gall bladder and stomach. This heat will soften and expand the tissues. The oil will permeate them and will penetrate the walls of the gall bladder and dissolve the stones; not at once, of course. In addition, drink half a glass of pure olive oil. You will have to continue this treatment until there are no gall stones, or until they are so small that they will discharge themselves easily. Live on natural foods and you will get into a condition where gall stones will naturally disappear.

Olive oil dissolves gall stones and lubricates the tube that leads from the gall bladder to the duodenum, and once the larger stones have been eliminated to the duodenum, we have won the battle. From there they can easily pass on and out through the rectum. As to food, cherries are excellent; also radishes, especially horseradish.

Q. What do you recommend for an infected gall bladder?

A. Put as hot applications as you can endure over the organ. Then drink a half cup of pure olive oil. Heat will attract the blood, as well as the oil, to that region. After half an hour, do some gentle exercises: swing hands up and down, overhead, sideways—any· thing that will stimulate the liver. The exercise will work the oil and blood through the tissues, and the infection will all come out. Do this every night. The blood is the best healer imaginable. Heat brings up the blood; exercise works it into the muscles; and the blood takes the impurities to the kidneys to be expelled. Then you will be clean and purified and a well man again.

GAS

Q. What will relieve gas in the system?

A. There is non-fermentable food, and also fermentable food. All cooked foods are fermentable, and some raw foods also, especially in wrong combination. Onions and garlic, for example, will ferment, as well as nearly all fruits and the raw cereals. Notice, however, that uncooked food ferments are sweet, whereas cooked foods give you sour ferments. The latter are injurious, but the sweet ferments are merely annoying. There are some strictly non-fermentable foods; namely, roots—such as potatoes, carrots, and turnips—and herbs, like lettuce and spinach. Eat these non-ferment-

able foods and you will soon clean out the phlegmy
condition that causes ferment. This phlegm once put
out of the system, you will not suffer from any more
gas.

Q. My wife is troubled with gas accumulation
which causes great distress. It sometimes lasts an hour.
These attacks come on whenever she has mental shocks
or fright, sometimes in the morning from two to four
o'clock, when her stomach is entirely empty. What
would you recommend?

A. I would find out what natural fruits, leafy herbs,
and roots she likes best. After she has lived on them for
some time she will not be filled with gas. I would teach
her corrective psychology, to help her fits of fright.
The reason she gets them is because she is so negative,
so sensitive that she will jump at almost anything. All
this also helps to cause gas, because many important
nerves center around the stomach. Cooked foods will
ferment, eggs will decay, and milk is a natural ferment
because it has been exposed to the air. Have her eat
natural foods instead, some nice fruit juice at breakfast
time. Find out what herb she likes best. If lettuce, give
her some lettuce and honey at noon. The lettuce is rich
in iron and will pass through the bowels without disturbance. Give her all the lettuce she will eat so
that the bowels will discharge the phlegm with the
lettuce waste. As the process of the peristaltic action
on lettuce will probably create gas at first, it should be
eaten in a coarse state so that it will be mingled as little
as possible with the phlegm and will act as a scraper
in the stomach. Gas is derived from phlegm. When

there is no phlegm, there is no gas. Vegetables, except those in the onion family, will never cause gas; neither can the roots. They will clean out the phlegm from the bowels.

Q. Do you maintain that those having gas can rid themselves of it by eating greens and raw food when it is a recognized fact that they give gas?

A. Gas, when you get it while on 100 per cent live food, is caused not by the food but by the accumulation of phlegm it stirs up. This gas helps to move the bowels, through which much of this phlegm will be expelled.

Q. Would gas in the stomach cause a person pain under the shoulder blade, in the region of the heart, and what is the cause?

A. A mixture of fruits and cereals, or nuts and vegetables, cereals and nuts, or the eating of dairy products: anything to make gas, or phlegm which will change into gas, must be avoided. When you want to overcome a gaseous condition, you must adhere strictly to a mono diet. That means you must find the one kind of food you like best for a particular meal, and eat it alone, without anything added to it. When you eat oranges, eat them alone. When you eat a head of lettuce, or carrots, or radishes, eat them alone. Gas pres· sure has been known to not only give pain, but also to stop the heart.

Q. What is good for one who has gas on the stomach after each meal and belches gas each time that food is taken into the system?

A. If you eat live food, do not blame the food. Keep it up until all the phlegm is gone. A raw potato every day with your roots will help out very quickly, but do not chew it very fine. Swallow it as coarse as you can. These "chunks" will clean out the phlegm. Continue this until you know your stomach is clean. Nothing will do that more thoroughly than little "chunks" of potato, apple, carrot, or rutabaga. Eat only two meals a day, at noon and in the evening.

Q. What is a good treatment for the elimination of gas bloating of the stomach?

A. Belching is good for taking away the pressure. When you cannot belch, drink warm water. That will open the pyloric valve and cause gas to pass out through the bowels. There are many effervescent preparations to cause you to belch, but do not take them. They are all salt compounds and are dangerous. If there be gas in your system, it will have to come out either by belching or by way of the rectum. Under all circumstances, encourage elimination of phlegm. Cold applications will compress the abdominal region, forcing the gas out by way of the rectum or esophagus.

GOITRE

Q. What would you advise for goitre?

A. Three things: clean out your body and keep it clean, do the seven neck exercises I shall mention, and use compresses. As to the last named, put applications around your neck, three times hot alternating with three cold. Keep the hot applications on twice as long as the cold. The hot applications bring the blood. We must produce a hyperemia in the region of the goitre. Then do the seven neck movements: 1. Move head backward and forward seven times. 2. Swing head straight across from side to side, seven times. 3. Bring head around from one shoulder to the other, likewise. 4. Hold your face straight forward and turn it to the left with a quick jerk, and then to the right with a quick jerk. 5. Drop head forward, then swing it from left to right, in a clock-like motion. 6. Same, only in opposite direction; both seven times. 7. Drop head forward as far as possible, bring back slowly as far as you can, and shake it sideways. Remember to do these exercises after the hot and cold water applications.

Q. What is the cause and cure of goitre?

A. There are two principal kinds of goitre. One is caused by bad habits, together with bad eating; the other is caused by nervous trouble—the thyroid gland being enlarged in both cases. Every disease can be traced to incorrect diet, so, as a cure, eat those live foods which you like best. Also use hot and cold applications on the neck, and do the seven neck movements. That will improve the circulation in the thyroid gland, and it will soon be reduced to its proper size. If the above treatment does not cure the goitre rather quickly, then make a mash to help soften this growth, as it may be fibrous. The mash is made from bitter almonds and sweet almond milk. Put this on every night before you go to bed and every morning upon arising. It must extend entirely around your neck. That will soften the fibrous tissues, but remember, you must be living 100 per cent on natural foods. Fasting on alternate days is sometimes beneficial. There is no need for an operation.

Q. What foods are best for goitre?

A. Since the thyroid gland is ductless, working by the influence of magnetism, Nature's remedy is the root food, roots being magnetic. All underground roots act magnetically and aid the magnetic functions of the body. Therefore roots, like the carrot, beet, turnip, even horseradish, will, if you like them, do your goitre a great deal of good.

Q. Should iodine be used in goitre cases?

A. Many think they must use iodine for enlargement of the thyroid gland, called goitre. That is a mistake. Inorganic iodine, such as you buy at the drugstore, is a poison, and the bottle containing it will be so labelled. Organic iodine, of course, has considerable value, especially when not combined with inorganic substances such as salt. You should get your iodine in the uncooked foods your taste calls for. Very little of this element is needed to keep the body in tone.

GONORRHEA

Q. What should be done for a gonorrheal infection of the eyes?

A. The same thing as for any other disease—clean out your body. In addition, put lemon juice in water and use as an eye wash, to cut the phlegm. Also use it as a rubdown for the whole body, and internally as well. Your entire system needs to be cleansed, for the gonorrheal condition is not only in your eyes, but throughout your body. Get plenty of sunbaths, exercise, and sleep. This is the only natural and correct cure for all diseases. Be persistent.

Q. Will live food alone cure gonorrhea?

A. Gonorrhea is a putrefactive disease. Though confined to local parts of the body in its early stages, the symptoms gradually spread. This disease is susceptible to the same treatment as any other disease, and is not any harder to cure than certain chronic diseases I could name. As often emphasized, live food alone will not cure anything permanently—you must prepare for and consolidate your victory by eliminating injurious habits, whatever they may be, and build up instead routines of action which are in accordance with Nature's laws. This means sunshine, fresh air, sleep, exercise, constructive thinking, and other beneficial practices.

GOUT

Q. Is gout curable?

A. Gout is a constitutional disease caused chiefly by the deposit of uric acid and urates in the body tissues. All acids are painful, and uric acid is not the least of them in this respect. The alkaline urates have a crippling effect, but in themselves cause little discomfort. The favorite location of gout is in the big toe. However, you will find it less frequently in the palm of the hand, the wrist, or the finger joints. The alkaline urates find lodgement in the tubercles that hold the ends of the muscles to the bones. Due to the contracting effect of these urates upon the muscle ends, you will soon find the joints twisted out of shape in a more or less permanent way. Sometimes you see the big toe twisted up out of alignment, or two or three fingers; even the back. You may have seen people hobbling about by the aid of two sticks. These unfortunate persons have gout deposits between the vertebrae of the spine. That makes it impossible for them to straighten up.

The cause, in most instances, is the eating of meat, associated with plenty of salt. The remedy, as usual, is to live steadfastly on the natural foods you prefer. You may have to train your tastebuds a bit at the beginning, since you will find that many foods which at first you do not particularly like are really very delicious after you have eaten them for a while.

Use alternate hot and cold applications on the affected regions. Then manipulate your joints by stroking and rubbing. Pull and twist them, rotate them one way, then another. Double them up and back. Put them into an all-night poultice made of ground raw onions and potatoes, half and half. Put this mash on copiously, so as to fully cover the joints. Every morning when you take off the poultice, again use the hot and cold applications and do the massaging, twisting, and pulling I have just spoken of. Get plenty of sunshine on your body, direct, not through glass.

GRAINS

Q. Is wheat food for humans?

A. Wheat is not food for man; it is for animals which have gizzards, and man has none. The bird has a gristmill in its body, called a gizzard. Inside this are pebbles of rock and gritty substances which grind up the seed and get it ready for the stomach. If we were meant to eat wheat and other grains, we would have a gizzard also.

Wheat has been advertised to death. Commercial companies have prepared wheat in many different ways for the sake of becoming as rich or richer than their competitors. They are extremely anxious that you believe wheat to be an excellent thing for man to eat, that it will cure this and that disease. It will not—it will, rather, bring disease, even that disease called cancer.

Q. Will you please tell us why grains are not good foods?

A. In the first place, all cereals have a tendency to ferment. That is a real disadvantage. However, if you will eat them uncooked, you will find them fairly good subsistence material, although acid-forming. Oats can be chewed very nicely, and corn is a fairly good food also. Corn is easily masticated when made into a coarse meal. The objection some people have to eating oats; namely, that they are a little bitter, may be overcome by eating them with honey. We have a nourishing dried sweet corn that is prepared while it is yet in its fresh, soft state on the cob. The kernels of corn are taken off the cob while the corn is still in the milk state, not too ripe. Then the kernels are dried in the sun so as to retain the sugar and prevent molding. Wheat, on the other hand, is very hard to handle. If you eat wheat at all, you should eat it raw and dry, and should masticate it thoroughly. Chew it until it becomes glutinous. It is only then that you will get any real nourishment from it. Exposing it to a heat of 350°, as in baking, destroys the value; even 160° or 200° F. produces the same result. All meals should be ground as close to the time of consumption as possible.

HAIR AND SCALP

Q. What can one do for baldness?

A. There are various kinds of baldness, one being where you lose your hair only on certain parts of the head. This is brought on by giving the hair improper nourishment, or by wearing stiff headgear that does not permit nutrition to get into it. Such a hat presses the small veins that supply the rootlets of the hair, shutting off the nourishment. Many have starved their hair not only by wearing wrong headgear, but also by eating wrong food. Cooked food contains little or no nourishment. I have had many patients who were troubled with falling hair. I have had men who were as bald as billiard balls. After two or three months on my treatment, hair started coming, and now they can comb it. Nature brings back the hair by restoring the rootlet, which is composed of a shaft and root. In this root is a little follicle with a tiny vitamine at the end, just one one-thousandth of an inch in diameter. When this follicle is in normal condition, the hair will grow again. It furnishes the oil neces· sary for the hair, so that you will not have to add oil to the scalp. Eat correctly, and the natural oil will come from within.

One of the best treatments for baldhead is to stand in the sun, and with the fingers give the scalp some kneading and massaging. You may also pull your hair, if any—a very helpful thing. Just rotate the fingertips, press firmly, then rub the scalp loose, and pull the hair. Alternate this with striking your head gently with the fingers. The vibration method also is very good. Put your hands on each side of the head, fingers over the scalp, and vibrate them. If you want to know what vibrating means, put a pan of water on the table; then put the hands on the table. When you commence to vibrate your arms, you will see the water quiver. A vibration from the hand is the most normal vibration you can get, always in harmony with Nature, with vegetable growth, and all animal life. Do this faithfully every day. Wash your scalp at least once a week with a good vegetable soap that contains no lye, potash, or animal fat.

Q. Can you cause hair to grow by eating raw food?

A. Raw food is live food, and it will replenish the little hairs on the head and all over the body. Raw food has living cells that put into the blood the vitality to induce growth. In conjunction with eating in this manner, take your hat off. Throw it away, and let the sun shine on your scalp. Then, with some good vegetable soap, give the scalp a good cleansing. Get some crude oil, put it over your bald spot or pate, leave it on for about ten minutes, and then, with some of your soap, wash it off again. Next, let the sun shine on your head for about ten minutes. Do that once a week, and see if it does not improve the growth of your hair.

Q. What can be done to stop falling hair?

A. Falling hair is caused by dandruff, the elimination of the scalp. Wash the scalp with vegetable soap, kneading it thoroughly while the lather is still on it. After you have washed the soap out of the hair, take a teaspoonful of pure olive oil and rub in. Olive oil has the smallest molecule of any oil and will make it much easier for the dandruff to come out.

Q. What food is necessary for falling hair?

A. Cabbage, cauliflower, lettuce, spinach, carrots, turnips, and rutabagas.

Q. Please give method of treating loose dandruff.

A. Dandruff is usually loose. Massage your scalp well every day. Rub in olive oil now and then. If you are a woman and have long hair, brush it with a brush, one hundred strokes a day. Massage the scalp with the fingertips, rotating your fingers in so doing.

Q. What foods will produce a sturdy growth of hair?

A. Any food rich in calcium, particularly cabbage and turnips; also cauliflower.

Q. What is the reason for dry scalp?

A. Dry scalp is derived from lack of circulation. Here is a good remedy: put your hands on the back of your head, filling your lungs with air. Bend forward and back as far as you can several times. This brings the blood to the hair, nourishes the roots, and brings new moisture to the scalp.

Q. Please tell us how you keep your hair looking so well.

A. If there is any part of my body which gets less consideration than others, it is my hair. In my morning shower, my hair always gets wet, yet it does not seem to suffer. When I get through with that, I comb it back and forget about it. One of my daily dozen exercises is especially good for the hair. This is it: I put my hands on the back of my neck, hold my breath, and bend forward several times, down as far as I can get. This brings the blood to the scalp. I never wear a hat, for sunshine has a stimulating effect on the hair follicles.

Q. What can be done for scabies?

A. Many babies are born with scalp disease called scabies, or milk crust. This is not natural to the child —we must blame heredity or wrong living. Nature never makes a mistake; Nature is always true to her principles. Therefore, the person who violates natural law demonstrates that truth by exhibiting such things as disease in his children. Scabies or milk crust may show up as a chronic disease, but if the child starts living on natural foods, its body will be cleansed and eventually this condition will disappear. The best way to treat any scalp disease is to take care of the body. Give your body the best of care and you will have given your scalp the best of care, for the scalp is a part of it. Eat natural, tasty foods. See to it that you have plenty of fresh air, bathing, and plenty of exercise. In the case of an eldery woman suffering from scabies, I prescribed very rigid exercise, as well as fresh air, sunshine, and bathing. She was to take a one-hour sunbath every day between nine and eleven, exercising at the same time until she was moist with perspiration. She was then to go into a warm bath, as warm as she could endure, to stay in it fully half an hour with progressive heat, which means increase according to endurance; then she was to get out and rub off with cold water. She had fruits in the morning, herbs at noon, and roots at night, and at the time of her third treatment, in the third week, she was practically well.

Q. What causes the hair to become gray on a young person of thirty or thirty-five? What is the best remedy?

A. Wrong eating, general abuse of the body, as well as, in some cases, heredity, are responsible. As for remedy, first of all eat live food. Eat plentifully of foods rich in chlorophyll, such as spinach, red beets, olives, strawberries, and blackberries — all the fruits and vegetables that have a dark, rich color.

Here is a helpful exercise that will bring nourishing blood to the roots of your hair: put your hands together, palm to palm, put them back of your head, take a deep breath, and bend forward as far as you can, holding your breath until you feel the blood rushing to your face. Straighten up, exhaling as you do so, take one or two deep breaths in an erect position, and repeat the exercise several times. If you are old and feeble, all you need do is to lie on the bed with the feet up and your head down, until your face gets red. Then get up. Do that twice a day, and it will not be long before your grey hair disappears. Massaging the scalp, too, is always helpful. Do this with your fingertips.

Q. Is dyeing the hair ever justifiable?

A. Do not put any chemicals on your scalp, for very often they contain poisonous ingredients that will make the remedy worse than the disease. Do not believe all you see advertised. Depend upon natural methods and you will come out right.

Q. How can one remedy split hair?

A. It may be due to the hair becoming unduly hard, similar to what happens in hardening of the arteries. Do you eat white sugar, salt, and other condiments, or cooked food? If you do, you are eating the same things that cause gall stones and hardening of the arteries. You may also be using a very astringent soap that causes the ends of the hair to become brittle and break.

Q. Do you consider hair dressing injurious to the hair, and if so, what would you advise to keep the hair in place?

A. If you have plenty of natural oil, you will probably not need any hair dressing, but if you have very dry hair, I would suggest that you first wet your hair with water, take about a thimbleful of pure olive oil, and work in while the hair is still wet. You might try a small amount of orange juice in place of the olive oil.

Q. Do our bodies lose in strength when the hair is cut?

A. Biblical history tells us that Sampson found it to be so. Be this legend or strictly accurate fact, some people have reported that they have felt a decrease in vital energy after their hair was cropped. There is some basis for the assumption by analogy with radio reception, the hair serving in the same capacity as antennae wires; namely, to intercept the aerial vibrations and transmit them to the nervous center, thence to the rest of the body. In the absence of definite measurements of these subtle forces, however, little more that is positive can be stated at the present time.

Appearance is a factor in mental peace, and that, or its contrary, reflects upon the general health of the body. This is something to be taken into account when there is a question of wearing, say, long hair, when everyone else cuts his short. Beards are out of style. It is an open question as to whether man does not lose considerable vital force by daily close shaving. Women, to my mind, have benefited considerably by the introduction of short hair as the vogue. Often headaches could be traced to excess weight of hair on frail persons; this, to be sure, while the body was living under unnatural circumstances.

HALITOSIS

Q. What should I do to get rid of a foul breath?

A. First of all, see that your teeth are clean. Foul breath often comes from hollow teeth. Go to the dentist and have them filled. Take care of the teeth you have. They are better than store teeth. Never let anyone persuade you to have all your teeth pulled to get rid of your disease. That is rank folly.

Furthermore, get your stomach and bowels clean through the eating of uncooked food. Constipation and halitosis usually go together.

HARDENING OF THE ARTERIES, TISSUES, AND GLANDS

Q. Will you tell us the proper treatment for arteriosclerosis, as well as the cause?

A. Arteriosclerosis is hardening of the arteries, a disease caused by eating foods full of inorganic minerals. These are such substances as come from the earth —salt, Epsom salt, baking soda, borax. The human body is incapable of digesting these inorganic substances, hard as it may try. Just as salt, dissolved in a glass of water, recrystallizes after a time, so in the body, being as unaffected by digestive juices as by water.

Therefore, when you eat salt with meat or potatoes, it soon recrystallizes in your joints and body tissue, hardens the arteries, impeding the blood circulation. What happens when these arteries get hard and brittle? When a rubber tube is fresh and new, it is elastic, pliable, but let it get hard, and what occurs when you try to bend it? It will break. Try to bend a glass tube; it will snap. Just so with your own arteries and veins when they get inelastic. Then you have what is called an attack of apoplexy. This generally takes place in the brain, since that is where these blood carriers are most subject to the salt hardening. When you are excited, or overjoyed, or excessively worried, the blood rushes to the head and suddenly dilates these veins. If they are hard, they may break. You fall over, unconscious. Sometimes the heart fails, a very critical condition, and traceable to the eating of crystallized salt. You can eat sodium chloride by the pound if you get it in organic form, as in spinach, beet tops, celery, or other vegetables, as well as fruits, but never eat it in crystallized form, for then it will inevitably kill you.

Another thing that helps to bring on arteriosclerosis is the high protein of flesh foods, generally salted, of course, to make them go down more easily. High protein is the cause of high blood pressure, too, and in the body's effort to throw off protein poison, danger of a blood vessel rupture is greatly increased. You are thus doubly likely to have apoplexy.

When you have once abstained from salt and flesh food and switched over to natural nourishment, you are half way along toward recovery. A few miscellaneous pointers follow: be careful to avoid excitement. Again, if you are quite old, you should wash your scalp once a week with a good vegetable soap; then apply some olive oil to soften the tissues, but do not massage the scalp at first—just rub the oil in gently and let it penetrate. After a month you may start massaging in the oil. Also give your scalp a first-rate rubbing every morning.

Q. When there is a swelling or hardening in the cervical region, due to lymphatic glands, what can be done?

A. Stop eating salt. Stop taking inorganic minerals into your system. Be careful also about what kind of water you drink, because sometimes much mineral matter is put into the body in that way.

HAY FEVER

Q. Is there any specific cure for hay fever?

A. Confine yourself wholly to fruit juices and raw vegetables. To break up an asthmatic or hay fever paroxysm, practice the following: throwing the head back as far as you can, inhaling, and blowing out through the mouth. That gets your chest up far enough so that the lungs can expand to their fullest extent without lifting the ribs. The sufferer from hay fever has weak lungs which are full of phlegm. He should practice long, deep breathing. This liquefies the air. Then let him cough out the phlegm.

Q. What is the cause of spring hay fever?

A. Poison in the system that needs to be burned up.

HEADACHES

Q. Please state cause of headaches located at top and back of head. What organs are involved, and what is the remedy?

A. The venereal and rectal organs are involved.

Take a hot sitz bath for a half hour and cool off with a cold cloth. Exercise the pelvic organs by lying on your back and rotating the legs back and forth. These movements take in all the muscular tissues of the bowels, the bladder, and the rectum. They will cause the blood which the heat brought there to be absorbed. Be sure to have the water as hot as you can bear it. Keep it so until the very last. If you find a slight dizziness coming on, put a cold cloth over the forehead or neck, or take a glass of cold water and sip it. Do this every night.

Q. When I do not drink my morning cup of coffee, I get a terrific headache. How can both coffee and headache be eliminated?

A. Barring temporary dislocations in the nervous system, also eye strain, etc., the majority of headaches arise literally from the sewage afloat in the veins. Your body is filled with the long-accumulated poisons of dietary abuse, which, stirred into activity by the natural foods you have been eating, are seeking an outlet by way of the eliminative organs. This usual type of headache does not attack you until some time along in the forenoon or early afternoon, since during the rest period of slumber the organs just mentioned can handle even the excess waste without being noticeably overburdened.

Why not try a day's fasting, with only lemon juice in plenty of water? This will give your system a chance to concentrate on the work in hand; that is, on the cleansing of the body. On the day after the fast, you should again eat, and you will doubtless find that your headache, though reappearing, will have diminished in intensity. On the third day fast again, on the fourth eat, and so on until your object is achieved.

Q. Immediately before or after the menstrual period, I invariably suffer from headache. What causes it? This, though I have been a strict live-fooder for two years.

A. Headache and stomach disorders in these cases often go together. Watch your diet carefully. Eat sparingly, or, better yet, not at all, during the first day, and the second if necessary. You very likely are still eliminating rather heavily, but, in time, doubtless the need for unusual caution will cease. During the menstrual period, obviously there is an excess of mucous in the bloodstream, overloading the eliminative processes, resulting in that signal of disease, headache.

HEAD NOISES

Q. What should one do for noises in the head?

A. Get rid of your catarrh. Stop eating dairy products and all types of cooked flesh. No catarrhal condition can be cured as long as you eat foods that are decayed or fermented, which include milk, butter, cheese, fish, eggs, and meat.

HEART DISEASE

Q. Please give diet and exercises for valvular heart trouble in a child.

A. He should eat the uncooked food he likes best. It may be apples or oranges in the morning, lettuce at noon, and possibly carrots at night. He may have flaked nuts with his morning fruit, and flaked peanuts with the lettuce and the roots. Use, say, a half ounce of nuts to begin with, and gradually increase the quantity as desired. Remember, valvular heart trouble primarily comes from uric acid in the blood. The patient should eat natural foods, take Epsom salt baths and deep breathing exercises, and the valvular heart trouble will yield wonderfully.

Exercise is very essential. Here are some move· ments: inhale slowly and deeply, putting hands over head; then hold breath and bend forward, touching first one knee, then the other. Also bend straight forward after inhaling, holding the breath meanwhile.

Q. Can leaking heart valves be cured, and what diet is best?

A. Yes, leakage of the heart can be cured, but as the cure depends somewhat on exercise as well as on diet, you must eat properly for at least six months before you can undertake the exercises. Thereby you will have sufficiently improved your blood and gotten your heart strong enough for the vigorous muscular movements which are necessary to cause the heart tissues to absorb new blood and to cleanse them thoroughly.

Valvular leakage of the heart is caused by excess uric acid, waste matter. The principal uric acid foods are meat and fish. Flesh food contains fourteen grains of uric acid to the pound, livers contain nineteen grains, and sweetbreads seventy grains to the pound. These waste products, when eaten, give us more uric acid than we can eliminate, and when it stays in the system it destroys the corpuscles of the blood. This brings on rheumatism, neuritis, heart disease, and much else. There are other so-called foods that contain no uric acid but substances that act in the same manner; namely, tea, coffee, chocolate, also cholocate candy. Coffee contains caffeine; tea contains theine and tannin; cooked chocolate has heavy theobromine. All these substances are just as bad as those found in flesh and fish.

If you want to cure heart leakage, you must stop eating and drinking all these, and live one hundred per cent on natural foods. The strawberry is the fruit rich· est in earth salts. It will give you blood that has rich color and the greatest amount of energy and dynamic force. Your blood once in good condition, you should exercise, which will cause it to flow faster through the heart.

Q. What can be done for weak heart valves?

A. We can strengthen them. Heart valves are simply tissues that can be easily stretched out of shape if you do not keep them continuously strong with organic tissue salts. To do this you must have good blood, eat natural foods, and get away from the exciting environment which may so easily snap the thread of your life short some day. Get away from city life; get out where there is little excitement and plenty of sunshine and fresh air. Mild exercise is very beneficial.

Q. Will you please give a remedy for a lady past seventy who suffers from a pain in the heart? She was ordered by a doctor to remain very quiet. She is also troubled with constipation and is very weak.

A. Yes, all in this set-up go together. Constipation produces toxins, toxins bad blood, which in turn causes the heart to get weak. When the blood is continuously pumped through the heart, the heart muscles are constantly saturated by that blood. If you eat food that is clean, pure, and full of life and energy, which will clean out the old blood and give you new, is it not possible that the heart will be restored again? What shall this patient eat? First of all it is necessary to discard all dairy products and flesh food, which includes fish. Instead, the diet should consist of uncooked vegetables and fruits according to taste. They will build blood and flesh.

Q. In cases of heart disorder, such as murmur, palpitation, etc., are hiking and sunbathing harmful?

A. Do not overdo them. When the heart commences murmuring, reduce your walking speed. I would change my gait and also my method of breathing at once, in such a case. Take slow, deep breaths to help oxidize the blood. Get a drink of cold water. Wet the forehead and mouth, and take some more long, deep breaths of air. If that does not relieve you, get someone to give you a concussion over the second and third vertebrae. The heart will stop murmuring immediately. As to changing your gait; if you are walking slowly, walk faster. If you find that makes you dizzy, swing into long, slow strides, breathing slowly and deeply at the same time.

Sunbaths are not harmful providing you are eating natural food, but if you are eating cooked food, be very careful about the vibrations of the sun, because they are not congenial to dead tissue. When you have created blood and tissue from dead flesh, and from cooked vegetables, there is no affinity for sunshine in your body. Wear a hat, and place a cabbage leaf under the crown. This is to keep your head cool and away from the direct rays of the sun. Also drink cold water. Wash your face and hands in cold water, and, if you can, wet yourself all over. You should not absorb too much sunshine.

Sometimes people think they are suffering from heart trouble, when it is really gas on the stomach. There is a fluttering or palpitation of the heart due to pressure of gas from below. The proper treatment in this case is to get rid of the gas.

Q. How shall one treat inflammatory rheumatism where the patient's heart is weak?

A. When there is a fluttering of the heart, put hot applications in that region to bring in an abundance of blood. Of course, the blood is full of uric acid, the basic reason why the heart is weak, but put on a hot application just the same, alternating with cold, until you feel that the organ is commencing to beat regularly again. This may have to be done many times, especially at night when the patient is asleep and he gets a fluttering of the heart which seems to take his breath away. To get good, rich blood, eat Nature's food, uncooked. Then watch your heart improve also.

Q. What is the cause of a weak, "fainting away" feeling around the heart, as well as a smothering feeling when you lie on the left side?

A. If you get the catarrhal phlegm out of your lungs you will not suffer from that smothering feeling. It is the phlegm that your lungs, also the digestive tract, are filled with, that makes you desire more air. You very likely do not have good blood. To remedy that, eat foods rich in phosphorous, like apples, raisins, almonds; and turnips and radishes, which are rich in sulphur. Your system needs stimulation. Take one tablespoonful of horseradish, grated, and mix with the same amount of flaked peanuts. Put a teaspoonful of raw flaked peanuts into your mouth; leave on top of your tongue. Then add to it some of the mixed peanuts and horseradish, chew, and swallow. The peanuts will prevent excess irritation. Eat the entire quantity prepared. About half an hour later you will commence to realize there is horseradish in your system. It will act as a stimulant and also clean you out. Do this every day.

Q. I am troubled with a pain in the region of the heart. It is excruciating when I walk rather fast upgrade or lift anything heavy. What is the remedy?

A. Apply hot applications whenever you have a pain. Give yourself a warm bath, too, and let the water get gradually hotter until it is up to the endurance point. Remain in this for about half an hour; then take a cold bath for a few minutes. Do this once every day. Put the hot application over the spot where the pain is located, and keep it on until the pain stops. The inrush of new blood to the region is what does the trick. Eat live food.

Q. What is angina pectoris?

A. Angina pectoris, also called sternalgia, paroxysmal pain, or spasmodic aneurism, is a breast affliction. It is caused by a peculiar enlargement of the aorta, or large artery, which comes from the heart, forming a bag on one side, where you feel intense throbbing at times. This is accompanied by spasmodic pains in the breast and a peculiar feeling of suffocation. It is a disease that is tormenting, but not necessarily fatal. All cases of angina pectoris are to be treated from a different viewpoint because they are combined with dissimilar complications. Some may be associated with aneurism, pangs, and pains, as well as obstructed breathing, resembling hay fever or asthma. This last is of catarrhal origin, meaning too much phlegm in your blood. Phlegm comes from fermentable foods. All cooked foods are fermentable; therefore eat one hundred per cent live material. No medicine in the world can cure catarrh. Only food with life in it will do that. Eat natural raw foods and you will not have any trouble.

Q. I have eaten a good deal of meat during the course of my life. Would there be any connection between that and the valvular leakage of my heart?

A. Certainly. The excess of uric acids found in meats and fish, including liver, sweetbreads, and other animal organs, will cause leakage of the heart as well as rheumatism. As a cure, simply get away from the uric acid food, and this includes candy, tea, coffee, and chocolate. Eat natural vegetables and fruits in abundance. If you do this, you will have at first an unpleasant surprise—all the salts deposited around your heart valves and in the joints are going to become acid once more, as they dissolve. You may say that the oranges you eat are creating your rheumatism, or heart flutterings, but they are not. It is the stored-up acid in your system. Keep on eating the fruits and vegetables you like best. After one week, be sure that you take Epsom salt baths, because these foods are going to work the waste matter to the skin, and when you bathe thus the acid waste will be drawn out. Lie in the bath ten minutes; get out and rub off; then go back for another ten minutes, sponge off again; and so a third time. Do this every other day, and when you have found that you feel better, twice a week, and, after a time, once a week for two or three months.

Q. What is the best cure for fatty heart?

A. For one day eat the live foods that you like best; the next two days live on liquids—fruit juices and water; the third day you eat again, three meals, as if there were nothing wrong with you; then fast two more days on liquids. Keep up this sequence for two weeks, and your heart will offer less complaint. Live on natural foods all the while, for your blood must be vigorous and vital to cure your heart condition.

HICCOUGHS

Q. What is the best way to stop hiccoughs?

A. Hiccough is a spasmodic inhalation suddenly arrested by an involuntary closure of the glottis. The little daily occurrences of mild hiccough come from overeating, overdrinking, too much booze, or smoking, but usually are easily overcome. Break up that vibration of the involuntary action of the glottis and you have it conquered. Here is the way: take a glass of water and drink ten swallows while holding your breath. This is effective in nearly every instance.

In some cases, hiccough cannot be stopped in this way, since the involuntary muscles have become uncontrollable. These hiccoughs are not of the ordinary kind, not as strong, but run along as though one were trying to catch one's breath and not being able to do it. This is the kind that is dangerous. In this case, there are only two remedies that I know of: one is the magnetic wave, and the other is fasting. Keep away from food until the hiccoughs stop. That may be three or four days, but do not eat until then. You may take a glass of water now and again, but keep away from solids.

A person living on natural foods will never have a severe attack of hiccoughs, because this food keeps the organs in perfect harmony with the vibrations of earth, water and sunshine. When you eat natural food, you get vitality and strong tenacity that will make you forever immune from the chronic, fatal hiccough.

There is still another method sometimes used. Place your fingers immediately under the ribs, close to the pit of the stomach. When you get your fingers well under, bend forward over them. This pressing up against the diaphragm changes the vibration.

Another useful way is producing a concussion over the first dorsal vertebra. Put one hand over the patient's forehead, and with the other hand strike that vertebra. Do that in proper rhythm for seventy-five, ninety, or one hundred counts. It will jar the whole nervous system, and the hiccoughs will stop due to the change of vibration.

Be sure you go on a natural diet in order to remedy it forever. Natural foods will quiet and stimulate your nerves, each in its proper turn. Apples are good for the brain, especially the cerebrum, the reasoning portion. Lettuce is good for the noon meal, very soothing to the nerves. It induces them to rest and relax, which is what you require after a morning of hard work. Your evening meal may be of carrots, mixed slightly with green onions. This will induce sleep. Sleep gives your nerves rest, to recuperate and strengthen.

HONEY

Q. Don't you think honey was made for the bees and not for human beings?

A. If the bees made honey for themselves alone, there would be tons of it wasted every year, as they cannot eat it all. Also, if we did not eat it, the wild animals would. Bears are very fond of honey, and possibly other animals as well. It is nectar gathered directly from the flowers, and is not essentially changed by being carried and stored by the bees. Milk, on the other hand, is far removed from the grass which the cow fed on.

In cases of bronchitis, asthma, hay fever, and tuberculosis, few remedies are more useful than honey; also in cases of cancer. Honey will, as it were, pull the phlegm right out of you. You may eat it as it is, if you care to, or it will mix well with any other natural food.

Q. Is the rapid sugaring of honey a proof of its purity?

A. No. It signifies only richness in sugar quality. The honey brought here from Idaho and Oregon is very readily sugared; the fruit blossoms there must have a greater abundance of sugar than those here. Nearly all of our local honey comes from mountain sage and orange blossoms, and will last, sometimes, two years before crystallizing. Both the northern and southern honeys are pure; one is merely richer in sugar than the other.

Q. Is strained honey adulterated?

A. No, not necessarily. Honey, either adulterated with water or gathered too "green," will sour in a short time. If any other sugar, like molasses, is put into honey, it will stick to your teeth and betray its presence in that way.

Q. What food value, if any, has the comb in comb honey? Is it harmful to eat?

A. There is no harm in it, although it is not food. If you eat it, it will merely pass through you as so much bulk.

Q. How may one be sure than honey is unheated? Is not all strained honey heated in the extracting from the comb?

A. Heating seems to be a general practice. A dealer who should know, once told me there is no unheated strained honey, and there is reason to believe he is right. To be sure, honey is not necessarily heated to a very high temperature; merely to facilitate its extraction from the comb. Therefore the honey need not be damaged, implying careful handling, however. When your taste is once up to par, you will be able to distinguish between that strained honey which has been severely heated and that which has not. The flavor will be immeasurably better in the latter case. Why not eat honey directly from the comb? That is the only practical way of assuring yourself of the maximum in flavor and healthfulness.

INDIGESTION

Q. Is it advisable to proceed with the raw food diet when the digestion is very weak?

A. Of course. Raw food digests from one to two hours faster than cooked food — for that matter, is the only food that does digest. Cooked food merely clogs up the organs and ferments, while its so-called "digestion" takes place only by chemical changes, whereas real digestion, on the other hand, is by assimilation and absorption.

Q. What food and exercises would you recommend for one who has slow digestion?

A. Eat live foods faithfully. Furthermore, exercise will aid digestion. When, after you have had your dinner, you go out into the yard and do some hoeing or other work, you will aid the stomach in digesting the food you have eaten. It will digest in about one-half the time that it would otherwise. Of course, if you have no garden and have leisure to do some exercises, try these: clasp hands palm to palm, and swing them back and forth in front of you about fifty or seventy-five times. Or you might do side swinging movements, which are slightly more vigorous. You may also swing the hands up and down, and bend at the same time. These movements are all good. They help digestion by aiding in unloading the food that would otherwise stagnate the bowels.

Q. Is bicarbonate of soda harmful to take when one is troubled with gastritis?

A. I should say so! Bicarbonate of soda is a salt, and its continuous use will cause cancer, cataracts, hardening of the arteries, and arthritis. The salt gets into the joints and twists them out of shape.

Q. I am a live fooder, yet I sometimes have indigestion. Can it be due to overeating and complex mixtures, or are there other causes as well?

A. An automobile engine will choke and "die" under an excess feeding of the very best gasoline, as well as under an excess feeding of "wildcat." In the same manner, the human stomach can be overloaded with the very best of food, overloaded to such an extent that the power of digestion will become weakened, leading later to severe gastric disturbances. Humans, particularly those of the more active type, are expressly built for the necessity of an occasional and, under primitive conditions, involuntary fast. In this era of superabundance, it is necessary to restrain the appetite occasionally by exercise of will power. That is true markedly in those people inclined to be nervous and mentally active by temperament. These, due to their habit of expending large amounts of energy, consume a large amount of food. The necessity for such expenditure, however, not being constant, while the appetite does tend to remain so, the system will find itself flooded with food elements, just as the automobile engine with the best of gasoline. A periodic fast day, then, is entirely within the bounds of an intelligent scheme of life. There is much truth in the old saw: "We dig our graves with our teeth."

In regard to complex mixtures, I can only repeat that the best mixture is no mixture at all. Nature herself has furnished, in each of the fruits and vegetables with which she presents us, a perfect combination of elements. If apples alone do not satisfy you, try some grapes, or tomatoes, or oranges, and at your next meal, if lettuce alone is not enough, try celery, cabbage, watercress, or a simple combination of two or several of these.

INFANTS—CARE OF

Q. Is it right to keep a newly born baby unfed for three days?

A. No. Just because Nature has given the baby enough nourishment to endure three foodless days without suffering, is no reason why we should compel it to wait. The baby should be fed as soon as you can get it to take the nipple, and as often as it shows the inclination.

Q. Do you recommend corals for teething children?

A. When baby gets a little older and wants to

chew, do not give him a rubber ring or coral, but a carrot. A rubber ring is not food; it is made out of processed sulphur. Coral is also unnatural for the baby to bite on, and is not good for him.

Never give a baby a rubber nipple, either. He wastes his saliva; is, in a way, being fooled by the substitute article; and having the nipple in his mouth is very unnatural. If baby cries, there is a real reason for it. Study his needs and care for them—don't merely silence him and allow his needs to remain neglected.

Q. Is it safe to raise an infant from the first without clothes and with plenty of cold baths?

A. In temperate weather, there is nothing better for a child of whatever age than exposure of its skin to the air and sun. A zero wind is a different matter; even fur-clad animals seek shelter in leafy burrows and nests. Man, perhaps, was intended by Nature to live in semi-tropical latitudes, whereas the more energetic find themselves penalized for their migration northward by being compelled to wear protective coverings of an artificial nature. However, the stimulating nature of the climate of the north, when combined with proper natural food and sufficient out-of-door exercise, tends to equalize matters.

Therefore, I should say that a child should wear the minimum of clothing necessary. Some of the healthiest children known go barefooted practically all winter in the latitude of Minnesota. As far as exposing tiny infants to extremes of temperature, direct sunshine, and the like, are concerned, it is reasonable to suppose that Nature would have them acclimated grad-

ually—direct sun for a few minutes at first, increasing
the amount from day to day. The same is true of
exposure to the air without covering; meaning by air,
the natural, unheated variety. Cold baths should also
be cautiously introduced, allowing for gradual adapta-
tion of the organs to their new environment.

Q. Do you think that most infants are "made too
much of," always being watched, and fondled, and
disturbed? Isn't this bad for the baby?

A. Certainly. Under natural conditions, the child,
after the first few months, would be left increasingly
to its own devices, to contacts with others of its own
age, rather than to those with adults. Unfortunate
complexes have been traced by modern psychologists
to unwelcome attentions of adults. Self-consciousness,
irritability, lack of initiative, are all traceable to early
pampering by parents and others. A child should not
be tossed in the air, bumped on knee, patted, kissed,
and the like. This stimulates excessively the emotional
nature of the child, which should remain dormant until it is more mature, except for the instinctive reaction
of dependence upon the mother during the period of
nursing. Even masturbation has been traced to this
undue fondling. With the passing of time, the child's
dependence on its mother should become less and less.
A child is not a toy, but an embryo human being, and
should be respected as such. Do not watch over a
child as a cat does over a mouse. Hedge it in from the
most obvious dangers; foresee the others insofar as you
are capable, and your own nerves will be more relaxed,
and the child much happier.

INFANTS' DISEASES

Q. What causes a nursing child to have colic? What is the cure?

A. Colic is caused by the mother's wrong diet. As to cure, put the baby on its stomach, roll it a bit, and the gas will pass off. The mother must live on live food.

Q. What causes summer complaint? Can it be guarded against?

A. The cause is, here as elsewhere, unnatural living, on the part of the child and its mother. The prevention and the cure are obvious. If the mother's milk were of high quality, there would be no trouble of this kind. But what with cigarrette-smoking, rouged mothers, how can a child be normal? Cows' milk, in cases where mothers do not nurse, is constipating. Elimination in such instances would be acute and painful, often resulting in death. Moral: Avoid unnatural milk. Use the juice of ripe oranges and other fruits and vegetables, freshly prepared. Have you ever tried watermelon juice? It is mild and nourishing.

Q. How can one eradicate a rash covering the face of a tiny infant?

A. Very young infants often have a rash to heighten their already ruddy complexions. Pimples in adults and rashes in children have the same cause—namely, poisons in the system finding a vent through this medium. Apply no powders or salves, but get to the root of the matter—improper feeding.

JOINTS

Q. What causes the synovial fluid in the knee joints to dry out?

A. The eating of salt, vinegar, sugar, and cooked food. Put hot applications over the joint until it is red; then exercise. Extend the hands in front of you; bend knees far down. The blood will work in, and soon you will be able to do the bend without a cracking noise. This blood will furnish the necessary lubricant.

Q. What is the proper way to treat a knee joint that is sore when walking, but not at other times?

A. Put hot compresses over the knee, to induce the blood to come into the area. When red, put a cold cloth over it. Now some exercises: do the knee bend several times, or until you get tired. Do this every night before you go to bed.

Q. What food would you recommend for making stiff joints loose and flexible?

A. Natural foods will give you natural lubrication, but they alone are too slow. You must give your joints hot baths or compresses every night for half an hour, and after that a quick, cold sponge. Then exercise these joints vigorously. The hot applications bring the blood, and the exercising forces the muscles to absorb it. This new blood softens the tissues. When your joints are hard, try bathing them with nut milk.

Q. I have a severe pain in certain parts of the left knee every time I touch it or do exercises. The doctor told me the X-ray showed foreign material present and the only way to cure it was by operation. What do you advise?

A. You will never get well by an operation; it may cause a dry joint and permanent stiffness. Dip your knee into a vessel of hot water; hold it there as long as you can, say, twenty minutes or half an hour, until your knee gets red with blood. Then take it out and put it into cold water, until the skin feels cool. Afterwards, move your knee by doing exercises, such as bending up and down. That will cause the blood you brought there to be absorbed into the tissues, which is what we are after. Remember, nothing heals like your own blood, and for good blood you must have live food. Practice this bathing and exercise every morning and night. It is well to take Epsom salt baths at least once a week. Get plenty of sunshine on the knee—twenty minutes at first, then thirty minutes, and keep on until you can leave it in the sun for an hour. Never sit still in the sunshine if you can help it, but exercise the entire body.

JUICES

Q. Please tell us how to preserve grape juice.

A. The juice is best preserved in the grape itself. Pack in moist sawdust and put in a cool place not subject to changes of temperature.

Q. Can carrot juice, or any other vegetable or fruit juice, cure cancer, as some have claimed to have accomplished?

A. Very true. Cancer may be attacked by the carrot juice method, and very likely other juices as well.

Any live food will carry on the good work of expelling waste and building up anew. There are, however, some foods which are better than others for this purpose. Whether carrot juice is better than the carrot itself, is an open question. True, you can drink more "carrot life" in the form of juice than you can eat in the form of carrots. On the other hand, it is also true that many juices are unnaturally prepared. They should, like milk, be extracted by the mouth directly from the source—the fruit or vegetable itself. Expectorate the pulp if your stomach rebels against it. When cancer is in the digestive tract, or near it, juices are of great value, and irritation will be avoided by their use.

Q. Under what conditions is the juice of a food better than the fruit or vegetable given us by Nature?

A. First of all, in the case of infants at weaning, and even somewhat earlier; secondly, where stomach and intestinal irritation must be avoided.

Q. Is there danger in taking juices exclusively over a period of time?

A. Juices, as I have often stated, are not entirely natural foods, especially when exposed to the air for some time before drinking. Moreover, the body requires bulk to keep the intestines in good working order. Prolonged juice fasts are dangerous. My system of alternate-day fasting, with fruit juices on the fast days, is safer and better.

Q. Are not pressed juices in a state of fermentation, being exposed to the air while being prepared?

A. When properly prepared and chilled, they will

keep sweet for a considerable time—at least a day or two, under favorable conditions. Fresh-pressed juices, made daily, are in all cases preferred where juices are desired. Fermentation under such conditions seems negligible.

Q. What is the relative merit of carrot, celery, beet, rhubarb, spinach, parsley, apple, grape, and coconut juices?

A. You will be told that celery is good for the nerves, the beet for blood-building, the coconut for energy, and so on. This, in general, is true to a certain definite degree. However, under no circumstances should you eat or drink a food which your tastebuds do not call for. Try a food, if you are told it will help your condition. Then, upon repeated trial, if your taste-buds rebel against it, have nothing to do with it. It may be food for others, but not for you, at the time. If your tastebuds do call for a certain natural food, and doctors or dietitians tell you it is not especially good for your particular condition, don't worry—follow your instinct. Nature never makes a mistake, but humans do. Even though a food is not especially rich in the certain desired element, you can easily eat enough in time to do the work necessary. On the other hand, it is easy to overload the system with an undesired quantity of certain elements, which must then be a burden to the organs of elimination.

KIDNEYS

Q. What would you advise for stones in the kidney or bladder? I have lived on raw food for a year, but frequently pass small stones when urinating.

A. When you have stony substances in your digestive tract, you need oil. One of the best lubricants is
olive oil. It has the smallest molecule and will penetrate any membranous tissue in the body. Use plenty
of oil with your food; just as much as you can manage
to enjoy. It will penetrate through the avenues of the
veins, digestive circulation, the tubules of the gall
bladder, the pancreas, the ureter (from the kidneys to
the bladder), and if there is any sign of a stone or
systoid growth, it will be dissolved. If there is any
unnatural substance present, it will be lubricated so as
to pass out quite naturally.

Q. I have a pain in the back, a sharp, shooting pain,
which seems to be in the region of the kidneys. I
should appreciate it very much if you would tell me
how to cure it.

A. If the pain is sharp and stinging, you very likely
have an ulcer. You must reach it as quickly as possible.
One way is by lemon juice, in the course of digestion.
Drink the juice of half a lemon two or three times a
day, nothing else with it. Apply a hot pad or hot water
bottle in the region of the pain for half an hour. Then
take the heat pad off and rub yourself dry with a cold
cloth. Next, do as many exercises as you can, without
causing other pains. The healing process will go on
in that area where the pus growth is located until the
pus is finally eliminated in the form of a boil or carbuncle. Be persistent, and you will be rid of your
trouble. Nothing heals better than your own blood,
but be sure your blood is pure from right eating.

Q. I have had an examination of my urine, and the doctor says it contains crystals which indicate Bright's disease. What can I do for this?

A. The best remedy for Bright's disease is the one which you like best selected from the following list of foods: tomatoes—the tomato is often called the kidney cure because of its wonderful healing value; then comes the cucumber—in kidney trouble, the cucumber is not far behind the tomato in worth, and is better for washing out the kidneys than is the tomato; watermelon is very good, as are other melons, like cantaloupe, honeydews, Persians, casabas, Japanese. Raw spinach and beets are also splendid, as well as raw Spanish peanuts. Roots are not particularly good for diseased kidneys. The oblong variety of cranberry is worth trying.

Q. What does a faint trace of albumen in the urine indicate? Is it a forerunner of kidney trouble?

A. Not necessarily. If you have eaten plenty of eggs, it may be that some albumen will pass through with your urine. That is really a good sign—you get rid of the egg albumen in this way. Other foods, too, send albumen to the kidneys—flesh, for instance. If you eliminate this through your kidneys, consider yourself fortunate. Do not continue to eat albuminous foods; your kidneys will be overworked, get weak, and finally not be able to function normally.

Q. What is the cause of kidney trouble? Water runs through in about forty minutes.

A. The first thing for you to do is to cleanse your

kidneys. Then the best remedy in the way of a food is watermelon. Eat watermelon for breakfast for about a week. Other foods of value in cases of kidney disease are tomatoes, cucumbers, the various melons, and raw peanuts. You have overworked your kidneys by eating high protein foods, such as meat, fish, and eggs.

Q. I have very tender and sore spots in the region of the kidneys, mostly on the right side. There are some traces of albumen.

A. Put some hot applications on that side, as hot as you can bear. Keep the hot cloth applied for half an hour. You may use an electric pad instead if that is more convenient. Keep it on for half an hour or until you get relief. This will bring up the blood, which will carry off the waste matter and do the healing.

Q. What is the relationship between kidney trouble and the eating of flesh?

A. Meat, containing an excess of uric acid, tends to break down the kidney cells through overwork in excretion. The kidneys are equipped to handle only a small fraction of the amount taken into the body daily by even the most moderate meat-eater. To be sure, the kidneys can, under stimulation by the glands, work at a feverish rate for some time, but sooner or later that will have to cease. Then the penalty for long-continued abuse of the system will have to be paid for, in coin of suffering.

LIVER

Q. Please tell me what causes liver trouble and how to cure it.

A. Liver trouble is always caused by eating cooked food. Cooked carbohydrates overwork the liver and clog up the entire system with toxins, bringing liver trouble and gall stones in their wake. This last named disease comes through the saturating of the liver by salt, which process gets the organ so large, finally, that it cannot function. Fortunately, we have a remedy: namely, olive oil. Take up to a half cup of it at a time. Use only the best, and you will find it delightful to the tastebuds. It will cure the liver and dissolve gall stones.

Q. Will you please tell me what can be done for an enlarged liver?

A. Enlarged liver is due to unnatural circulation resulting from wrong eating. When you feel any distress, take a half cupful of olive oil. That will permeate all outlets of the liver and help it to eliminate its secretions. Live on natural foods throughout; avoid salt eating, as this makes the liver into a storehouse for waste matter. Use plenty of olive oil with your food.

LONGEVITY

Q. How long should humans live?

A. Human beings have gone a long way toward self-suicide, but very little toward maintaining and prolonging life. The oldest man was Methuselah, according to Scriptural records, and he lived to be nine hundred sixty-six years of age. According to the same records, there was no one between Adam and Noah who did not live well over three hundred years, many as long as seven or eight hundred years. Now, why should we not live two hundred years? An Oriental, by the papers, is reputed to be two hundred fifty years old. I myself would gladly live to be five hundred years old. If we can remain healthy and strong all that time, who would not want to do the same thing? We know that all animals but man, in his perverted state, live from seven to ten times their average age of maturity. For example, a horse is mature at three, and lives to be thirty or more. A man is mature at twenty. According to the same ratio used in the case of the lower animals, he should live, at the very minimum, one hundred and forty years.

Q. In your opinion, what are the chief causes for the short span of life of the human race?

A. I am daily struck by astonishment, not because humans do not live longer than they do, but that they continue to eke out year after year of even a precarious existence. I wonder at the long sufferance of Nature, how, driven into one corner, she will escape into another, from thence to another, battling always against extinction of life. True, the amount of vitality in the average body steadily diminishes, until in middle life the individual is indeed more dead than alive. He is a walking monument to death, the god whom he serves, pathetically, all unknowing.

Specifically, the greatest foes of longevity are the

cooked foods. Next after these rank lack of fresh air, sunshine, and rest; unhygienic clothing and dwellings, and the dissipation of vital powers in sex, overwork, and the like. It may be, too, that through long generations our vital powers as well as our bodies have been weakened, that we who have lived on cooked food until well along in years, cannot expect to live out the full span allotted to Methuselah, or even impart the possibility of that boon to our children and grandchildren. However, judging by the surprising comebacks made even in a few years of sane living, what to us may seem perfection may be arrived at within not too long a period.

MALARIA

Q. Can one so live that he will be immune from malaria in a malarial country?

A. Yes, I am immune from malaria, and you can all be so after you have lived one year on natural foods. People from northern climates go to the tropics and eat generously of pork, hot breads, and other foodless foods, drink much liquor, and wonder why they contract malarial fever. The body relaxes in the unaccustomed warmth and loosens a flood of poisons into the bloodstream. Proper diet will neutralize these and make them harmless, as well as any germ that may be floating in the air. The fruits and vegetables raised in the area, or close by, are the most valuable in every instance.

For an active case of malaria, fruit juices and water should be used exclusively until the fever abates, which will be within three to five days at the most. It is well to shield oneself from the malaria mosquito as much as possible, thus preventing an unnecessary burden upon the functions of the body in getting rid of the dead germs and toxins.

MASSAGE

Q. Is the masseur of use in aiding restoration of health?

A. For one thing, he is sometimes a diagnostitian. Let us say you have taken a course in massaging and that you are a full-fledged masseur. You massage five to ten people each day. Your hands are getting in touch with these different persons, and you begin to notice after a month or so, when your hands get accustomed to the work, that with one person you get a peculiar feeling in the head; with another, a face ache; with still another, pains in your side and legs, or some other part of the body. You wonder what that means. I shall tell you. When people are well, they have a normal vibration. When they are sick, they have a sub-normal vibration. Suppose you have a person under treatment and you begin to feel a twinge or ache in your head. You ask him if he has a pain in his head. He will look at you and inquire how you knew. You thus, by a kind of sympathetic attraction, are constantly learning the real seat of the trouble in each of your various patients. That is the way magnetic diagnosis works out.

For general diagnosis, you place the right hand back of the neck, between the two shoulders, and the other hand over the solar plexis. Let them rest there for a minute, and you will begin to sense the physical condition of that entire body. Regardless of whether the pain is in the toe or the skull, you will be able to shut your eyes and tell the individual just what the trouble is. You will not be able to do this until you have practiced massaging bodies, for massaging develops magnetism.

Q. In what abnormal body conditions is massage of value?

A. Massage is of value, broadly speaking, whenever there is undue tension in a certain part of the body, or throughout the entire nervous system. Massage has then a relaxing, a soothing effect, as in some nervous headaches.

When there is a congestion of blood in the stomach region, one's natural instinct calls for rubbing, which removes by pressure some of the blood attracted there, together with the poisons it has collected, making way for a fresh, clean supply. This is a case where massage is valuable for painful congestion. When there is congestion of waste matter, as an incipient appendicitis, the same would hold true. Massage will also make chiropractic adjustment more effective and permanent, due to the relaxation of muscular "pull" on the vertebra. Osteopathic practice may thus supplement the chiropractic.

MASTICATION

Q. Please tell us something about the mastication of food.

A. Thorough mastication is essential only for certain kinds of food. You do not have to masticate fruits, herbs, or roots further than is needful in order to swallow. But if you are eating cereals, you will be obliged to masticate them thoroughly. If you want to eat wheat, chew it until it has been turned into a gluten. (You can never get gluten from bread—bread is not the staff of life, but the staff of death. It introduces you to asthma, hay fever, and tuberculosis.) If you are constipated, swallow your fruits, vegetables, or roots in fairly large pieces, so as to furnish roughage for the bowels. That will mean plenty of sweeping material for the wastes in the intestinal tract, and will stimulate peristaltic action. Almost everyone suffers from constipation; it comes from eating dead food. Why? Because such foods do not encourage muscular action and your digestive organs have little work to do. The bowels, as a result, have developed no strength to throw off the waste matter, which means that you go to the drug store for a cathartic to blast it out. Eat live foods and you will not need any of these habit-forming pills.

Q. My stomach is weak. Should I Fletcherize my food in order to break up the tough fibres?

A. Some years ago Mr. Fletcher's method of mastication was extremely popular. Nowadays, however, his theories seem to have gone the way of all theories; namely, been supplanted by bigger and better ones. This is not a disparagement of Fletcher's contribution to dietetical knowledge, which is real, though perhaps slight.

It is obvious that large quantities of cooked meat and potatoes, swallowed hurriedly, will cause nothing but trouble. Smaller quantities of these, eaten in a more leisurely fashion, copiously ensalivated, would logically create less havoc in the digestive tract. But this method does not get at the root. Why is there here an urge toward rapid eating and over-indulgence? The system is starved for vital minerals, and above all, for the life resident in natural, unrefined food. The stomach has to go over a vast amount of cooked material to extract only a pitiful trifle of nourishment. To Fletcherize cooked foods, then, means that we furnish even less nourishment than before, because we necessarily eat less, although possibly the stomach may handle that diminished amount in a somewhat more effective way.

When we eat Nature's foods, unrefined and delicious, we need not think about ensalivating them thoroughly. The natural flow of the glands will take care of that. They will taste so good to us that we will unconsciously linger over the eating. Any tough gristles which may be in the food may be ground up by the teeth, or otherwise, only insofar as is necessary for easy passage down ward. In your case, however, you should be careful not to subject your delicate stomach tissues to undue friction. Simply avoid those things which irritate excessively, or, if you are especially fond of them, eat only a very small amount. Fletcherizing, in itself, apart from the grinding up fine of food particles, is apt to be injurious to the stomach rather than of benefit, since it is an unnatural thought-taking process, involving excessive stimulation of the salivary glands. Constipation, too, is made worse by the fact that scarcely any roughage is allowed to enter the bowel.

Q. Should food be mixed well with saliva before swallowing?

A. You won't be able to prevent it, provided you eat the right kind of food; that is, the natural food that appeals to your taste at the moment. It is well to keep in mind that a salad, though uncooked, is by far less natural than apples, pears, or grapes, juice-filled from natural ripening. Added stimulants, as in salads, are far inferior to the natural saliva stimulants found in well-ripened fruit, for instance.

MEAT

Q. Is meat more dangerous than cooked vegetables?

A. Meat contains the following amounts of deadly poisonous uric acid:

Beefsteak	. .	14 grains of uric acid per pound
Liver		19 grains of uric acid per pound
Sweetbreads	.	70 grains of uric acid per pound

Uric acid is a waste naturally thrown off in the regular course of activity from your body. Your system, in a normal condition, will create and throw off three grains in twenty-four hours. When you add to it by eating a pound of beefsteak each day, you will, in spite of emergency efforts on the part of the kidneys and other organs, get a surplus amount of uric wastes stored up in the tissues and elsewhere. Then come, in ominous procession, blood acidity, rheumatism, high blood pressure, hardening of the arteries, insanity, paralysis, cancer. Yet big billboards say meat is a health-building food!

Uric acid is the cause of ninety-five per cent of human diseases, according to Dr. Hague of London. Uric acid is the natural excess of waste products caused by metabolism in any body. It makes no difference whether the flesh is that of humans, or chickens, or cows, or fish—all flesh contains uric acid, about fourteen grains of it per pound. Cooked vegetables are acid forming and bowel clogging, but they do not contain uric acid.

Q. How can we get strong and develop muscle if we do not eat meat?

A. Grass furnishes all the elements for tissue building of horses, cows, or sheep. The sheep gets its food at first hand from Nature, but the human being that eats the flesh of the sheep gets it at second hand, plus the uric acid wastes. These uric acid wastes help cause rheumatoid arthritis. Furthermore, the flesh is not eaten as it comes from the animal, but with copious additions of crystal salt, pepper, ketchup, sauces, and other condiments. How many people would eat meat if they had to catch the animal, kill it, eat it warm, uncooked, and without seasoning of any kind? Yet that is precisely what every meat-eating animal does, with the exception of the vulture and other scavenger birds. If you should ever crave meat, just imagine you see cattle jammed into box cars, arrived at the end of a long, thirsty rail journey. The smell of the stockyards comes to their nostrils; the smell of blood tells them of their coming fate. They are maddened by fear. This fear poisons their blood and adds an extra amount of uric acid to it and to the meat which we later eat. Do you think this creates strength, or weakness and disease? Remember, the elephant is the strongest of living creatures, and he eats nothing but grains and vegetable products.

Q. The Bible does not seem to oppose the eating of meat. What is your opinion on this subject?

A. In a certain great Book we are told: "Have dominion over the fish of the sea, and over the birds of the heavens, and over every living thing that moveth upon the earth. And God said, Behold, I have given you every herb yielding seed, which is upon the face of all the earth, and every tree in which is a fruit of a tree yielding seed. To you it shall be for food." It did not say, You shall have dominion over animals to kill them. Suppose I had a section of land and on it some pure-bred cattle, horses, sheep, and chickens, and suppose I say, "My friends, you may live on that section of land; make yourselves happy there, and you may take charge of all the animals." Does that mean you may kill them? No, because every one that you kill would lower the value of my place. You would be stealing from me, unjustly destroying life. In the same way, you are stealing from God every time you shoot down a deer, elk, moose, or grizzly bear. You are taking something that does not belong to you—the life of an animal. "Well," you say, "I did it in self-defense." Perhaps you did, if it were a mountain lion or grizzly bear. But let us ask why they feel so very much afraid of you. You do not know? The grizzly bear has a keen

sense of smell, and at a distance of fifteen or twenty
feet he knows at once that you, if you have been living
on flesh foods, are dangerous, for your body will be
permeated with that odor. He fears you because he
believes you will kill him for his flesh. That is the true
interpretation. We have caused the animals to loathe
and shun us, even to kill us with their teeth and claws,
to protect themselves.

That may have been the reason Daniel, of the Biblical story, was not killed in the lions' den. He was cast
into their den, and the lions did him no harm. The
story says he had not eaten meat for many months, and
possibly never, so the lions did not even snap at him,
had no grudge against him. That may be the reason
why some people in this state have not been bitten by
rattlesnakes—the snakes will not even tune their rattles
for these persons. On a certain ten-acre ranch, the children have absolutely no fear of them; when they see
one, they herd it along, as it were. Once, on their way
to a neighbor's, these children, who had never tasted
meat, found a great rattlesnake in their path, and they
merely "shooed" it along. The snake put his head up
and went on obediently. When the children and reptile
were within a short distance of the house, the neighbor
came out to meet them. He was hardly in sight when
the rattler curled up ready for striking, and sounded
his warning vigorously. The children were alarmed,
but it was not they he was trying to keep off, but the
newcomer. They did not want the neighbor to kill the
snake, but the man refused to listen. When I was told
this incident, I asked if the neighbor ate meat. The
reply was: "Oh, yes, he always has a smoked ham or

a hind quarter of beef hanging in his woodshed." I
said: "That accounts for it. The rattlesnake knew. He
did not want to be killed by this meat-eater."

Q. Were you raised a vegetarian?

A. No. Let me tell you a story. A man had been
hired to paint father's new barn on our Minnesota
farm. He had only one arm. It amused me to see
how well he could handle the brush and ladder. When
he came to have lunch with us at the family table, I
sat next to him. I perceived that he did not take any
meat. Being of an investigating turn of mind, I took
notice, but did not say anything until after everyone
else had finished and gone out. Then I went to him
and asked: "Why did you not eat meat?" His reply
was: "Oh, meat is not good for anyone to eat." I wanted
to know why. This was the answer: "It makes men
wolfish." That was the exact expression he used. Of
course I was young and could not understand it completely, but just the same it made a great impression
upon my mind. He said that wolves tear up and
devour flesh, eat it, and then fight horribly with one
another. I did not say any more about it, only I never
offered him any more meat.

Years later I went to the Battlecreek Sanitarium to
learn their diet system. I noticed that they served no
meats. I had not eaten meat for many years on account
of that little remark of the one-armed painter, just to
learn how it would work with myself. Of course, there
was also something else that had helped turn me against
flesh eating. One day I had asked my father, who was
a doctor, whether meat-eating was the cause of rheu-

matism. He being a well educated man, I had great
respect for his answer. Sitting there at the head of the
table, he brushed his hair back and said: "Yes, I believe it is." I returned, "Why do you eat it? You have
rheumatism." He leaned over toward me with "Why,
you fool, because I like it." But I was not satisfied.
To myself I said: "Well, here is where I stop eating
meat," and I did so, although the temptation was a
frightful one for the next three weeks. So in the Battle Creek Sanitarium, while studying dietetics, I learned
that meat-eating was not only causing rheumatism,
but ninety-five per cent of the other diseases of man.

Q. Would a slice of tender ham be all right now
and then if I eat correctly otherwise?

A. At one time, when I was a young man, I was
a cook for a big threshing crew. It happened that there
was no meat on hand, and the farmer had to drive his
team of horses to town, fifteen miles away, to get some.
All the threshers, of course, thought their energy de-
pended upon the amount of meat they ate. When it
came, we in the kitchen commenced pulling the jackets
off the bacon, and lo and behold, when we did that we
saw that the meat was alive with maggots. One man
said that that was nothing, he would fix it. He put it
into a washtub, took it down to the river, washed away
all the worms, and sliced it. The men commenced to
call for the wormy meat, and ate it with great relish,
for the worms had put enough holes into it so that it
was beautifully tender. "What a man does not know
does not hurt him," it is said, but the law of Nature
is nobody's fool. You will pay for wrong living some

day, and in good measure. So whether the meat is tender or not, keep away from it.

Q. Is freshly killed meat harmful?

A. When an animal is dead, there is no life in it. That ought to be evident to anyone. We should not eat lifeless food. Besides, animal flesh will become gangrenous within twenty minutes after killing. It is bad enough to eat the flesh at once, immediately after the animal has been slaughtered, but you are often eating meat that has been on the shelf for eighteen months or two years. Frequently, this flesh has been washed in saltpetre water to kill the odor. There is a law in a mid-western state that no refrigeration plant may keep the same flesh in storage more than three months. There is also a law in an adjoining state to the same effect. So the packing companies of these two states, when the time limit has arrived, will exchange meat for three months. Then, if not all has been disposed of, they ship it back again. It is known that meat has been shipped back and forth in this manner for a year and a half. It then gets so tender you do not even have to cook it to eat it. In plain and simple language, it is rotten. If it has been freshened in a saltpetre solution, you think you are getting something very fresh and nice, but you're mistaken. In addition, the dried, exterior portions of the cuts are trimmed off by the butcher to give the meat a fresh appearance. And at times poisonous substances are used to color up stale cuts.

MEMORY

Q. What is the cause and cure of poor memory?

A. Here is one good way in which to cure a bad memory. It is an easy device, which, if consistently practiced, will aid in helping you overcome your memory difficulties. A simple case for example: A housekeeper who goes marketing should write down the various articles she needs on a slip of paper and put the list of items into her pocket. When at the market, she should try recalling as many of the articles as she can without referring to the paper. When she can think of no more, she may resort to the memorandum. Let her do this day after day for several months; then, if she has meanwhile been brightening the brain cells by eating live foods, her memory will be distinctly better. Soon she will be able to do all of her shopping without reference to any written list. Practice in memory training is of value in many fields: to the doctor in remembering the names and symptoms of his patients; the salesmen, his customers and their peculiar desires; the speaker, the proper sequence of his ideas, and so on. The library contains many books which go more deeply into the subject of memory-training.

Fundamental in all cases, however, is a clean body, which can be had only by vigorous adherence to the principles of right living. Children who, while living on cooked foods, had a very poor memory, have been known to become almost brilliant in this respect when they changed to a natural way of living.

MILK

Q. Why do you object to milk and its related products?

A. Milk was not intended for humans after they reach the age of eighteen months. Every child is born with a thymus gland, located in the throat. This gland is present only from the time of birth until it is eighteen months old. This is the gland which makes it possible for the infant to use milk as food, to digest and assimilate it. The sucking action of the mouth when nursing stimulates the child's thymus gland, which, thus stimulated, furnishes a substance which helps to digest the milk when brought into contact with it. Another thing—the milk is taken directly by way of the mother's nipple into the mouth, and from there goes to the digestive organs. No air gets at the milk at any time during the process. When milk is exposed to the air, you must watch out for catarrh, asthma, and hayfever—much phlegm will be produced in the system.

As to grown-ups, there is absolutely no excuse for their drinking animal milk. Cows' milk is for calves, and goats' milk is for kids. We knew a man who was the owner of a tuberculosis sanitarium near Long Beach which used the so-called milk cure. He often ate at our restaurant. I remarked to him one day, "I understand you are running a milk sanitarium." He replied, "Yes, we help them get fat." I asked him how long they would remain that way, and he answered: "Long enough to go home and get to work, lose it all, and come back for more." To the query as to whether they were curing many cases, he said: "Some people think we do, but we really do not." He was at least honest with me. Money to him, and others like him, is the prime end, not the true welfare of the patients.

Q. I frequently read statements that children who get plenty of milk make more growth, both physically and mentally. What do you say to this?

A. My experience has proved just the opposite. It shows that live food does not build fat, but muscle, bone, connective tissue, endurance, and mental vigor. Children who eat uncooked food, as a general rule go to the head of the class both in physical activities and in their studies. The calcium from orange juice is in every way superior to the calcium obtained from milk in its ability to grow a healthy child. Other fruits and vegetables contain a smaller, but very appreciable amount, of bone and tissue building material.

Every kind of dairy product is a ferment, one of the worst kinds. As soon as any such product reaches the stomach, it sours, causing lactic acid. This, in turn, changes to an alcohol acid, and no alcohol can digest; it is a fixed product. Therefore, the stomach churns it, works the alcohol into an ether, which can be gotten rid of only by evaporation. Milk taken directly from the nipple, without air having any access to the fluid, is good, provided it is mothers' milk and the child has not passed the age of eighteen months. The intervention of air brings with it bacteria and ferment, and hence the souring in the stomach.

Q. Is clabbered milk a good intestinal antiseptic?

A. No, instead it causes catarrh and all other types of phlegm diseases.

MINERAL ELEMENTS—INORGANIC

Q. Do you consider the injection of iron into the system harmful?

A. All injections directly into the bloodstream are harmful and unnatural. Food, tonics, and all sustenance must come into the body by way of the mouth and digestive apparatus in order to be mixed with the various fluids to be found there before passing into the blood. It is impossible for the body to assimilate inorganic iron, meaning the kind of iron you find in the drug store tonics and in the various mineral waters. In order for the body to make use of iron or other minerals, it is necessary that they be passed through and stored up in vegetables and fruits. If any inorganic iron should, by chance or otherwise, be lodged in the body tissue, it will act like a poison and will have to be thrown out through the kidneys, bowels, and other organs of elimination.

Q. Please explain the difference between organic and inorganic mineral salts.

A. Inorganic salt is taken directly from the earth in crystal form, and cannot be assimilated by the body. This applies to iron, sulphur, calcium, iodine, and the like, as well as the ordinary sodium chloride (table salt), and Epsom salts used as a laxative. Organic salts, on the other hand, are an ingredient in natural food, non-crystalline in form, and eminently suitable for replenishing the muscles and bony tissues.

MINERAL ELEMENTS (ORGANIC) FOUND IN FOOD

Q. What raw foods are rich in calcium? Are there any that equal milk in this element?

A. Spinach, cabbage, and the white turnip, as well as oranges and grapes, are rich in calcium. No, none are as rich in that respect as milk, but, on the other hand, calcium in cabbage and lettuce will not ferment; neither will that in the turnip, radish, or spinach. Milk, with its calcium, will ferment, because it has been exposed to the air. A baby must get its milk directly from its mother's nipple. If the mother can furnish no milk, it is better to give the infant fruit juices and nut milk, rather than cows' milk.

Q. Will you please tell us what function iron fulfills in the human body?

A. Inorganic iron tonics are very destructive to the teeth. Iron from lettuce is good for your teeth. Iron oxidizes the blood, thus burning up waste matter. It creates red blood corpuscles. People lacking a sufficient amount of it are anæmic.

Q. Would it not be better for one of weak digestion to take iron tonics than try to assimilate the iron in raw foods?

A. Dig anything from the earth, like Epsom salt, dissolve it in water, and if it goes back into the same form it had before it was dissolved, you can see at once that it does not change permanently. Many thousands of years are necessary for any change to be made in

mineral salts, except when they are absorbed into vegetation. When you find iron in the form of lettuce,
spinach, cherries, it is fit for human use. The plant
roots penetrate among the earth crystals. Then, through
the aid of sunshine, air, and water, these salts are dissolved sufficiently to make them available for absorption into the plant. There, other changes are made
which are necessary for their transformation into edible
foods for humankind. The proportion of the various
organic mineral salts to each other in the plant is what
determines the difference between the taste and value
of the plant, as well as its very nature. Each plant has
a certain proportion of practically every mineral element. The proportion may be large or small, but you
may be sure to find at least a small amount of iron in
practically every food plant.

MOUTH AND TONGUE

Q. What is the cause and cure of a bitter, burning
taste in the mouth?

A. The cause is improper digestion. To get rid of
the bitter taste, I would advise you to eat a dozen or
so dried olives after each meal and see how quickly
that will do the work.

Q. Will you please tell me the cause of a sore
tongue? I do not eat meat.

A. This irritation is sometimes caused by eating
certain natural acids that are too green, certain fruits
that are not ripe. Be sure your strawberries are ripe.
If you want to get a sore tongue quickly, eat a half-

ripe pineapple, or unripe fresh figs. Peeling one's figs often saves one's tongue much soreness.

Q. What is the best remedy for too freely flowing saliva?

A. Stop eating salt and sugar. Excessive salivation is often caused by them. A good way to overcome your trouble is to take some honey into the mouth, let it assimilate with the saliva, and spit it out. Do that once a day. In general, eat natural sweets, not cooked sweets, and eliminate salty and spicy condiments.

Q. What causes bad taste in the mouth, mornings?

A. Possibly you eat too near bedtime. You should eat three hours before retiring, and nothing, then, until morning. Cooked food may require all night to digest. Ham, you cannot digest at all, and when it does pass from you, it will have decayed to such an extent that it leaves a bad taste behind. Very likely your stomach is not in first-rate condition.

Q. My tongue is often coated. I take fruit juices in the morning, greens at noon, with olive oil and nuts, and roots with flaked peanuts at night.

A. Keep right on. Poisons are moving out of your system; that's all.

Q. How can one cure trench mouth?

A. Diseases like trench mouth come from eating canned food. The way out is to eat leafy vegetables, uncooked. For the mouth, I would recommend dried olives. Eat at least one or two after every meal; more if you like. They will probably make your mouth sore at first, but continue with their use, and eliminate the canned food.

MUSCLES AND JOINTS

Q. What causes creaking joints?

A. It is lack of lubrication. In watermelon time, eat your watermelon seed and all, the seeds to be swallowed whole. There is silicon on the outside of every seed, a wonderful lubricant for your joints. Moreover, the watermelon is an excellent cleanser for your kidneys. Put hot applications over your knee joints, or any other joint that creaks, every night before you go to bed, about half an hour on each joint. If it is your knees that squeak, do deep knee bending exercises several times after the hot applications. That brings the blood to the affected area. It will then, by means of exercise, be worked into the muscles and under the knee cap. This will create new synovial fluid in the joints.

Q. Is it necessary to have big muscles in order to be strong?

A. You know what happened to Goliath, the big giant who was slain by the sling-shot of the little Judean lad. Though this may not be exactly a test for strength, it does illustrate what often happens to the bulky contender for athletic and other muscular honors. The small man is apt to be what we call "wiry," with immense funds of energy unknown to his heavier rival. Here, in the field of muscle-building, as elsewhere, we should strive for quality rather than quantity. Uncooked foods build solid tissue; cooked foods, tissue that is more or less flabby. After you have been a live-fooder for some time, people will notice how solid your flesh is—legs, back, or biceps; it matters not where the test is made.

Q. Should a manual laborer do daily exercises for the sake of muscular development?

A. If he wants to be well developed in all parts of the body, yes. Very few jobs involve more than a comparatively limited number of movements, employing only a relatively small number of muscles. It is necessary for the fullest degree of health and vigor to exercise all the muscles in the body as far as possible. The exercises should, if feasible, be done before you begin your work, for afterwards the muscles used during the day, and tired out, will spoil your relish for what you are doing.

Q. What should be done for a shoulder thrown out of joint?

A. Put on hot water applications to ease the inflammation, this, of course, after you have gotten the bone back into its socket. In such cases, there is usually some attendant inflammation because of the sudden strain placed upon the ligament, resulting in injury to it. Avoid moving the shoulder any more than necessary, for a day or two. Sunbathing is beneficial, too.

MUSHROOMS

Q. Are mushrooms a healthful food?

A. Nothing wholesome can grow without sunshine, air, and water. That which grows in darkness is not food for man or beast. Mushrooms are a fungus growth, found in dark, moist places. Sometimes they are cultivated in cellars and caves. They are lacking in chlorophyll and practically all vitamines. In the stomach, they decay, instead of being absorbed and assimilated. Mushrooms should be avoided, whether formally branded poisonous or not.

NAILS

Q. What is the best raw food for growing finger nails?

A. Carrots, turnips, cabbage, rutabagas, are the best foods. Celery is also good.

Q. How can the nails and cuticles best be cared for?

A. The length of the nails as cut should depend upon the kind of work you are doing. They should not be too long nor too short, their sole function being to protect the fingertips from injury and to allow picking up articles with facility. Do not let the ends get ragged or broken; trim them off neatly with a file, a pair of scissors, or a knife. As to the cuticles, forget about them. Let Nature take care of her own beautifying. The cuticle has its purpose just as any other part of the body, and should be left undisturbed. The cuticle acts as a joining medium between flesh and nail. When the body is healthy, the cuticles and nails will be beautiful, as Nature intended, without any fuss or bother on your part.

Q. My fingernails split at the slightest provocation. How can I correct this condition?

A. Your trouble may be due to lack of silicon, the hair and nail builder. Eat those foods which are rich in this element: carrots, cabbage; also watermelon, including the seeds.

Q. Is manicuring, such as one gets at the beauty parlor, bad for the nails?

A. Mere trimming and polishing are legitimate enough, but no poisonous preparations must be used in the way of coloring matter or for heightening the lustre. Cuticle removers, too, should be taboo. If you wish to color the nails or increase their brilliancy, use natural vegetable or fruit products. You may be able to get these at reputable health food stores or at beauty parlors which have adopted the natural methods. You may have difficulty in finding one of the latter, and may have to be your own beauty expert for some time to come. Good red blood shows through the fingernails; they should not require artificial coloring agents.

NERVOUS DISEASES

Q. Please tell me how to cure nervous debility.

A. The nerves need better blood. Keep right on eating natural food. Be very careful that you always eat the food you like best. Eat just as much as you desire, within reason, and your blood will soon change for the better. It may take a year before you are entirely well, but use patience and good judgment.

Q. What should one do for nervous indigestion?

A. One who has nervous indigestion should seek a quiet spot, perhaps a little nook in the mountains, away from the hustle and bustle. There he will find sunshine, fresh air, and quiet. Wholesome natural foods are essential. Cut down somewhat on your intake of solids, and drink more fruit juices and water. If you eat carefully, and eat only a little at a time, you need not do any fasting. If that is not possible, I would then say you should eat only two meals a day, or perhaps one. If you care to try it, eat only every other day, with fruit juices on fast days.

Q. I should like to know what to do for a person whose hands and feet twitch and jerk considerably when asleep.

A. The nerves are exhausted. They want better blood. The blood is so full of toxins and waste matter that the nerves cause the disturbance. The person no doubt has cramps and pains. That is the natural reaction of the nerves when the blood is not good. The only way to get better blood is to live correctly. Spinach is the best blood purifier, the food richest in sodium and chlorine. If you like it, eat it plentifully, in its raw state, of course.

Q. Can neuritis be cured?

A. Certainly. The nerves pain you because they want better blood. When you live on natural foods, you will be furnishing elements that the nerves so insistently demand. Good, red blood is the best possible healer.

Q. What treatment is best for sciatic trouble?

A. The sciatic nerve complains because the blood furnished it is not rich enough in organic mineral salts and other food elements. In size, it is next to the greatest, the nerve in the leg. As a remedy: live on natural foods; take Epsom salt baths; practice slow, deep breathing every day. A prolonged alternating hot and cold bath every morning will also help considerably. Rub yourself with a stiff bristle brush to stir the circulation.

Q. What can I do for chronic sciatic nerve pain in the left hip? I have been living on uncooked food for about nine months.

A. Take a hot sitz bath, one just as hot as you can endure, or use a hot water bottle, keeping it on the sore spot for half an hour. Then immediately put a cold cloth over the hip for just a moment, and work your hip as much as you can. Lie on your back and move the hip this way and that so as to bring into play all the muscles in that region. The blood attracted there by the hot water will in that manner be absorbed into the muscles. The results from a few nights of this treatment will amaze you.

Q. Do you attribute the prevalence of nervousness to city life, with its hustle and bustle?

A. There is a vast deal of unnecessary noise in every city, which can easily be done away with by the adoption of sensible regulations rigidly enforced. The nervous system assuredly is subjected to constant strain in large centers of population, strain which is almost completely absent in smaller towns, villages, and on the farm. All the same, there is another side to the picture. Insanity, particularly among farm women, is a genuine problem in these smaller communities. The very absence of human sights and sounds often has an injurious effect upon the higher mental centers. Yet we may safely say that one who is nervously high-strung should reside, if at all possible, in a less active environment than that of our modern big city. For those who are obliged to confront noise, natural methods of living will be of immense benefit.

NOSE AND THROAT

Q. What causes tickling and soreness in the throat, and how should one treat it?

A. Tickling in the throat is always due to some phlegmy condition of the membrane, irritating you when you breathe. When the throat tickles, it causes you to cough. That is a good thing, although uncomfortable for the time being. Get rid of all the phlegm possible. If it does not come the first time, cough again, and keep on coughing until it does. Coughing is helpful, not harmful, when Nature finds it necessary to use that means to rid you of excess waste matter. The same is true of sneezing. When you finish you are relieved; no more irritation — the membranous tissues in the nostrils are clear.

As a fundamental cure for this state of affairs, keep

entirely away from milk, cheese, butter, eggs, and cooked foods in general, because these first named, especially, are phlegm producing and alive with aerial bacteria. At the time you drink milk, it may seem soothing to the throat, but it will actually add to the phlegm. Furthermore, the bacteria in the milk will feed on the phlegm in your throat. When they have eaten down to the live tissue, they tickle you and cause a still worse cough.

Live on fruit juices, watermelons, peaches, and other seasonable fruits. To about four ounces of chipped ripe avocado, add three ounces of tomato, and mix in some flaked almonds or pecans. There you certainly have something that will clean out old phlegm and not add to that which you already have. At noon time, choose something non-fermentable, like lettuce, cabbage, spinach, watercress, endive. You may mix these as desired; they are all good. For instance, take four ounces of lettuce, three ounces of flaked peanuts, and four ounces of rhubarb juice. Mix and serve. In the evening, try some roots. Take four ounces of carrots, three ounces of radishes, three of flaked peanuts, half an ounce of honey. Mix and eat. Don't eat or drink anything after you have had the last meal of the day. Have some orange juice before breakfast, and you may have another orange drink two hours after breakfast, if you care for it, and another half an hour before lunch. In the afternoon, drink vegetable juices—pineapple, for instance, or rhubarb. You may drink two hours after your noon meal, half an hour before the evening meal. Eat your supper and wait three hours before you go to bed; then the food will all be digested. Your stomach, as well as the remainder of your body, will be able to rest.

Q. What is the treatment for sore throat? Is permangenate of potash good?

A. This is an inorganic mineral, and you should not put it into your mouth, 'though you may bathe yourself with it, just as with salt water. The mouth should be considered sacred because what goes into the mouth goes into the bloodstream. Why not gargle with a little lemon juice, or the weaker, but efficient, orange juice, or grapefruit juice? If you want potash for your throat, why not take it in the organic form of dried olives? A little olive oil after the lemon juice will soothe any roughness that may be left there after the rinsing.

Q. After eating cucumbers, my sore nose commences itching. Does that mean it is beginning to heal?

A. Yes.

Q. Please tell me the cause and cure of nosebleed.

A. When you have been a live fooder for some time, you will never have nosebleeds. Why? Because your blood will have sufficient live sugar and salts to furnish the proper hemoglobin to the blood cells. As soon as any membranes get tender, the blood will cause them to thicken so that they will never bleed. Impure blood is due to eating devitalized material, cooked and valueless. Vito, or dynamic force, can be found only in uncooked foods in appreciable quantity.

Bleeding of the nose is not fatal. Though not considered dangerous, it is very debilitating, because you are losing life energy with every drop of blood. The first nosebleed of a series may not be bad, and probably you will not have another for six months. Then they may grow more frequent—monthly, weekly, and finally daily. At last you are alarmed and think you must do something. In an emergency case, take a little piece of absorbent cotton, fluff it up, and thrust it into your nose. Contact with the absorbent cotton should congeal the blood and stop its flow, but if not, your blood is poor in quality, lacks hemoglobin, and you will have to find something more active. There is a remedy which will stop bleeding under all conditions—cobwebs. There is something almost wonderful about cobwebs. No matter how large the vein or the artery which is cut, put a little cobweb on the wound, and the bleeding will stop quickly, like magic. Nosebleeds should be a warning. Commence to eat foods that will give you richer blood—live food, not dead food. Get away from the old routine of cook stoves, jellies, and jams, and the prepared foods you get in the grocery houses.

Q. Is honey good for sore throat?

A. Yes, it penetrates the inflamed tissues and loosens the phlegm. The blood then can circulate more freely in the healing process. Many times, however, sore throat is just a symptom of general elimination. In that case, too, honey will be of value, although naturally its main activity will be exerted elsewhere than in the throat.

Q. Why do I get polyps in my nostrils?

A. You shouldn't, if you are living on live food. That will clean them out in short order. Cooked starches produce them most freely.

Q. What is the cause of sore throat?

A. There are many causes, chief among them being elimination of poisons from the system by means of the respiratory passages. When the lungs are overburdened with waste material, some of it seeps into the throat, as it were, setting up an irritation.

NUTS

Q. Which is the most nutritious nut? Can we judge value by price?

A. The price is never regulated by the nutritive value of the nut. All nuts are good, nutritious food. Some, however, are richer in oil and carbohydrates; some contain more protein than others. Eat the nut you crave at the time.

Q. How many ounces of nuts, including peanuts, should be taken with meals by an adult and by a child, and at what time of day?

A. An adult may have about three ounces of nuts in the morning and three ounces of flaked peanuts at noon (of course, the peanut is not a nut). He should use peanuts also in the evening, for peanuts blend better with herbs and roots than do real nuts. Real nuts, on the other hand, harmonize well with fruits. Give a child who is quite young only about an ounce. An older child may have two ounces, and the grown-ups, three. If a child is fond of nuts, he must need them. Proteins are either destructive or constructive. If the nut you eat tastes delicious to you, it is doing constructive work. If it does not taste good to you, let it alone. Even those having good teeth often swallow quite large pieces of the nut. The nut is best eaten flaked, for more thorough digestion.

Q. Which nut may be eaten with vegetable salads at night when peanuts are not desired?

A. You may use pignolias, flaked, instead of peanuts.

Q. Which nuts, besides almonds, are not starchy?

A. All nuts are starchy. Everything that grows in fibre form, edible or not, contains a certain amount of starch. Some nuts, it is true, contain more than others —for instance, almonds are not very rich in starch. Brazils and cashews, on the other hand, have a great deal of it.

Q. Should one whose digestion is poor eat nuts?

A. Yes, they are good food when flaked and well masticated. If your teeth are poor, you will aid digestion by eating some dried olives before every meal.

Q. What is lacking in the coconut to make it a perfect food?

A. The element iron is lacking.

Q. Is nut protein ever harmful as flesh protein? Is it subject to the same putrefactive bacteria?

A. Nut protein should never be compared with flesh protein when speaking of foods, since nut protein is distinctly a natural food, whereas flesh protein is not. True, we can overeat on the best of natural things, thereby doing ourselves a great harm. It is particularly advisable to hold the daily allowance of nuts within strict limits, not so much because of the protein element as because of the nitrogen, a highly explosive substance.

As to bacteria, if nuts are eaten without being flaked or thoroughly chewed, there will be considerable putrefaction in the colon. However, this fermentation is of a sweet and non-destructive nature, while, on the other hand, fermentation of meat in the colon is sour and destructive.

Q. Do you recommend nut butter?

A. If your teeth are not good, nut butter will solve your chewing problems. However, remember that nuts can be flaked, which disturbs the cell structure less. In finely ground preparations like nut butter, the passage of time no doubt involves certain structural changes, making the food harder to digest, also less wholesome. No doubt Nature intended us to eat nuts from the shell, grinding them in our own "tooth mill." Therefore, if you want nut butter, purchase it freshly ground, just prior to using, or, better yet, make your own. There are nut butter knives for all standard makes of vegetable grinders. In the making of nut milks for infants or for use in raw soups, nut butters are preferable to flaked nuts.

Q. Are not all nuts acid forming? Why, then, do you consider them good food?

A. Eaten in moderation, they are a perfectly wholesome and beneficial food. In regard to foods, do not ask any other question but this: is it a natural food— that is, does it appeal to your tastebuds in its pristine, unrefined form? If so, don't worry about whether or not some medical chart labels it acid-forming or non-acid forming. You will have good results, provided caution and common sense are used. Although nuts can be eaten in combination with other foods, they are best digested when taken alone.

OPERATIONS

Q. Do you believe that operations can never do any good?

A. Never allow any surgeon to operate on you. In the first place, the various anaesthetics used, like ether and chloroform compounds, when taken into the body in the usual large quantities that are necessary to deaden pain and render the patient unconscious, have a more or less permanent detrimental effect upon the human system. The patient is seldom normal until six or eight months after the operation, and often not then. One of the symptoms which are commonly noticed after the operation is a derangement of the nervous system, an involuntary spasm or jerk of the muscles in certain parts of the body, coupled with a general lack of control. This, to be sure, is found mostly among those who eat cooked food. Their system is full of phlegm and consequently they lack power of resist-

ance against these powerful drugs. If you have had any
operations, be sure that you live on natural foods, for
they will help you to eliminate all vestiges of these
post-operation disorders by cleaning out the remains
of the inhaled or injected poisons. Natural foods will
not only restore the strength to your fibrous tissues,
muscles, and tender bones, but they will forever prevent operations by making you practically immune to
disease.

Q. Does scar tissue from an operation ever become
normal?

A. In case the operation was performed previous
to the patient's becoming a live-fooder, the answer is
"No." In case the patient is a live-fooder, the answer
too is "No," for no live-fooder will submit to an operation. Cuts, in one who lives on natural food, will heal
up with scarcely a trace to show where the injury has
been. Nature may thicken the skin just a trifle at that
point to make the ligature binding, but it will not be
the ugly white scar tissue so characteristically found
in others.

Q. Are not certain emergency operations necessary
in order to save life?

A. Ninety-nine per cent of all so-called "emergency" operations are unnecessary, beneficial only to
the surgeon and helpers. Emergency treatment of an
entirely safe and sane type is available for every
disease. Nature has her own remedy, and it is up to us
to discover and use it. As for the one case out of a
hundred, involving broken bones, etc., a competent

surgeon can be of great assistance, provided he does
not use harmful drugs.

OVEREATING

Q. Yesterday I had a distressed feeling, a kind of
seasickness. Could that be caused by excessive eating?

A. Yes, you can eat too much of anything, however
good it is, and you can drink too much, too. Some
people eat only one meal a day; in other words, they
eat all day long, but the stomach absolutely requires
rest.

Q. Is one overeating when he takes two pounds of
live food at a meal?

A. Never eat off a scale—judge by your tastebuds
and by the capacity of your stomach. When you have
a vague idea that you are not up to par, even on
natural foods, when these do not taste as good to you
as they should, stop eating for a day, also on alternate
days if the treatment is found beneficial.

Q. When there is a tendency to overeat on live
foods, how would you recommend that it be overcome?

A. You can use the aletrnate-day fast system; or reduce the number of meals eaten per day. Better still,
cut down the amount of food taken at each meal, without increasing the number of meals. In the last of these
three cases, you will find your stomach gradually returning from its stretched, inelastic condition, to its
normal size and resiliance. Then it will be able to
absorb much more nourishment out of a little food

than it formerly did out of a large "belly-full." Plenty of will-power will be necessary to break a habit of long standing, as overeating usually is. As a rule, this dates back practically to birth, always to adolescence, when the body makes tremendous efforts to get hold of body-building materials and finds very little in the average meal of cooked food.

OVERWEIGHT

Q. Will you tell us something about overweight and how to get rid of it?

A. Other names for overweight are "obesity" and "fatty degeneration." It means that fat has been deposited in the cells of the body. Fat, when found in a cell, is a superfluous substance, a normal cell being only about one-half or one-fourth the size of one of adipose, or overweight, tissue. The fatty condition may take in the entire body, or it may be localized in particular organs, or parts. There is a disease known as fatty degeneration of the brain; there is also a fatty degeneration of the liver, and of the nervous system. This last named sometimes proves fatal, for when fat cells insinuate themselves into certain nerves and nerve centers, they cause inflammation, depression, and inactivity. This is also true in connection with the lungs. Then there is also fatty degeneration of the heart. This also has proved fatal. Yet none are beyond remedy if natural foods come to the rescue, for these will not allow any universal or localized form of obesity to exist.

This condition comes about through foods that have

no adhesive tissue, a form of cement for the cell, a binder that holds the cell to its original size. Adipose tissue is abnormal, unnaturally large, as we have said. The best way to get rid of such a state of things is to eat natural foods, choosing from these always the ones you like best. Eat fruits in the morning—they are the best eliminators. Fruits will incur the expulsion of waste matter. Do not try to hasten the process of cure. Have no fear, for Nature is never dangerous. She knows exactly what to do in every instance if you will furnish her the proper materials with which to work. Mother Nature supplies the best food on earth, but do not spoil it. Though many cooks think they can improve on such food, the only time they seem to do so is when it is already spoiled. Cooks will take flesh which has a bad odor, wash it in saltpetre to destroy the taint, then boil it or fry it, and you wouldn't know, upon eating it, that the meat was really rotten. They will take spoiled flour, mix it with alum, and produce nice-looking white bread, so white that you could not detect any trace of the original material. Or they will mix a poor quality of fish oil with a high grade of olive oil, so that it will be difficult for even a good chemist to detect the imposture. Animal oil is often substituted for vegetable oil. All this is done by the "art" of cookery. The overweight person should have greens at noon, with flaked peanuts, and roots at night, with the peanuts if they are desired.

Q. When I have been sitting for a while and then get up, I have to stretch to get the crease out of my waistline. What causes this and what shall I do? When

I am tired, it is worse. I am a 100 per cent live-fooder now.

A. You are too fleshy around the waistline, and the fatty tissues there stick when they are folded together. You need plenty of sunbaths, Epsom salt baths, massage, and exercise. Mountain climbing is a good thing if done in moderation. Get the flabby flesh worked off and you will not have any more creases to bother with.

Q. What foods will reduce and at the same time give strength?

A. Every person has master builders in his body. These are the tastebuds on top of the tongue. The first thing you should do is to get acquainted with yourself and your real tastes. Ask your tastebuds what it is they like best in the raw menu. Do not dictate and say, "I want you to keep me in strength and at the same time reduce me," because the food is going to have its own way. Do not be alarmed; keep on reducing even if you get to weighing twenty or thirty pounds less than you ought to, just so that you become purified, for natural foods will not build flesh where there is a great deal of waste matter in the body. You cannot deceive natural foods; they must have a clean body. They will not commence to add flesh until the body is clean. There is no danger in reducing your weight so long as you live naturally. You say, "People talk about me." Why worry about that? They are not your friends, or they would not want you to eat that garbage again, misnamed "cooked food." The very best friend you have is your body. Take care of it.

PAINS AND ACHES

Q. What is the best thing to do for extreme pain in the shoulder and back of neck? I am a 100 per cent raw-fooder.

A. Any kind of pain is relieved by either extreme heat or extreme cold, heat usually being the more desirable. The heat brings the blood to the surface, where the pain is. Once the blood has satisfied the nerve that is giving you pain, you may put on a cold application, just cool enough to freshen the skin. By so doing, the blood will be driven off, carrying with it the toxins, and the tissues or bone will be relieved of congestion. Nerves call for blood through pain signals. Pain does not necessarily indicate an injury—it is merely a warning that there is something wrong. It is the ringing of a servant's bell, as it were, a call for action. So put on the hot applications until your skin gets quite red over the painful spot. That will relieve you. Then put on a cold application for just a moment or two.

Q. What causes pains in the hip, running down to the knee and foot? When I cough, I feel them more intensely.

A. There is some sort of acidosis there, neuritis, perhaps, following the nerve channel. Take a hot shower, let it strike the hip and run down the leg. Follow this at once with a hot foot bath, and then with a cold shower, and rub dry. Keep your foot in the water at least twenty minutes to half an hour, the water being as hot as you can endure it. Do this every morning, and, if your leg is very painful, every night as well.

Q. I have sharp, shooting pains in my back, under the left shoulder blade. Please tell me how to cure them.

A. When you get those pains, put a hot application over the spot, a wet cloth, as hot as possible. Leave it there until the pains are gone. The heat will bring the blood to soothe the nerve. When it has quieted, put on a cold cloth. Never massage a pain area, for you will only spread the inflammation, and, if pus is present, it will go all through the tissues. Help it concentrate in one center, and this will be the point of elimination.

Q. I have a pain in my left knee. What do you think is the cause, and how shall I treat it?

A. In the first place, put some hot applications on the painful spot. Then kick the leg out hard. Get the blood circulating throughout. Rotate the leg. Do whatever you can think of to get the blood going. Finish up with cold water packs for just a few moments. When once you have the blood circulating properly, you will be all right again.

Q. I have a pain between the shoulders. What would you recommend to cure it?

A. Get the uric acid out of your system by taking Epsom salt baths once or twice a week before bedtime. Take sunbaths, and put hot applications right where you have the pain. Remember, your blood, even though it is not very good, is the best healer you have. The hot applications are for the purpose of drawing it to where it is needed. The nerves will be pacified, and the pain recede as the blood carries away with it the toxic material. Finish up with a cold application for a moment or two.

Q. Please tell me how to cure a pain under the left shoulder blade.

A. Use hot applications, and you might need chiropractic adjustments, several times if necessary. If you know of a good chiropractor, ask him to examine your spine. There may be a lesion between the third and fourth dorsal.

Q. I have a pain in the neck at all times. What is the cause?

A. There must be some vertebral misplacement, or misadjustment. Try this: after massaging the cords of the back of the neck, let the adjustor place his right hand on one side of the patient's face and the left hand on the other side of the face. Then let him jerk the head to one side, then to the other. After this, proceed with the movements given for the cure of headache. Put hot and cold packs on the back of the neck. Do this every day, and the pain will soon disappear. Some say chiropractic adjustments do not help them. Many persons taking chiropractic treatments feel excellent results at first. Later, the old symptoms return. Often both the patient and the chiropractor wonder why.

Suppose you are operating an electric bell, with batteries. Ring that bell every day for a year and something is bound to happen—your bell battery will be exhausted. Some people's body batteries are exhausted in like manner. They then have not the dynamic energy within to be able to respond to the chiropractic release of the nerves. Live a natural life for a period of time and you will not need any chiropractic assistance. Learn to be your own doctor.

Q. What causes pains at the base of the brain and across the top of the head? These come early in the morning and never last through the day.

A. Pain across the top of head and base of neck is always an indication of trouble in the rectal region. Pain across the forehead indicates stomach trouble. Pain in the temple indicates eye and nerve trouble.

Q. What should one do for a general backache?

A. The most important thing is that you start living a natural life, and if you are already doing so, continue. By a natural life we mean proper live food, exercise, plenty of sleep, sunshine on the whole body, and fresh air. You may also try these exercises: place two chairs in front of you, a short distance apart. Put your hands on the chairs and bend down forward as far as you can. Then draw yourself back to the original position. Do that seven times. Then, in the same leaning position, swing one leg over the other and back again seven times. Do the same with the other leg. When you have done that, turn yourself around, face upwards, and do the same exercises, only in reverse, as it were. Do this every night before going to bed, and every morning on arising.

PALSY

Q. Please explain how to cure a palsy patient.

A. A palsy patient is one whose nerves are crying out for better blood. Live naturally and eat uncooked food—fruits in the morning, herbs at noon, and roots at night.

PARALYSIS

Q. What is the treatment for paralysis of the arm?

A. Paralysis is generally caused by one of three things: toxemia, malnutrition, or some parasite, like a tapeworm, that takes away the nourishment from the body. Try to find out first which of these it is. You can easily discover if there are any worms in your system by examining the excrement, and whether or not you are toxic by the complexion and the condition of the blood. If you are eating cooked foods, you may be sure you are adding toxins to your body every day. When the body has come to such a pass that paralysis has set in, you are in a bad way, but nevertheless there is still hope. Remember that when nothing else on earth can cure you, live foods always can. We know that live foods have certain vitos which give off a vibration conducive to the creation of new energy, especially when you are in the sunshine, exercising. By and by the muscles will become normal again; you will feel an impulse to do something, a little more each day. Eat natural foods just as they are indicated by your own tastebuds—fruits in the morning, herbs at noon, roots at night; and after you have lived in this manner for about three months, commence to give your arm definite treatments. Produce hyperemia in the muscles that lead to the hand by alternating hot and cold applications. Then rotate the hand to cause the muscles to absorb the blood; afterwards the shoulder should be manipulated in the same way.

Q. My husband, who had high blood pressure, suffered a stroke of paralysis about a year ago. Can anything be done for him?

A. Feed him natural foods; cleanse his system with Epsom salt baths twice a day (morning and night), bathing until clean. He must have a bowel movement as many times a day as he has meals. Get him into the sunshine between the hours of nine and eleven each day, about fifteen minutes the first time, twenty minutes the next, and so on, until he can stay out for an hour. Get him to do all the physical movements he can. If he can move any part of his body, let him do so until tired—all this while out in the sunshine. While nourishing his body in this manner and through eating vital foods, he will be able gradually to renew the nerves that are seemingly dead. When the motor nerves will apply their energy to the muscles, the body will become mobile again. It may take anywhere from one year to five years, but have him stick to it.

Q. What will cure creeping paralysis?

A. Natural foods correctly chosen, with exercise, sunshine, and water. Always eat the natural food that you like best.

Q. Is there a disease known as plastic paralysis? If so, is it curable when it is destroying the brain cells of a five-year-old child?

A. Yes, it is curable. Natural food stops the destruction of the cells, especially of a child, and, given time, renews them once more.

Q. Will the raw food diet cure infantile paralysis? I have a boy twelve years old whose right arm has been paralyzed since he was a year old.

A. A raw food diet, together with the water treatment I shall explain later on, will do it. It is the quality of the blood that makes or eradicates disease. Raw food replenishes the blood, and this, when directed to the affected area by hot and cold applications, will work a permanent cure. Infantile paralysis is a disease of the cerebral-spinal column. Put the hot applications wherever the disease has centered. Continue until a great deal of blood has been drawn there. Then put on cold applications and massage on each side until the blood is worked into the muscular tissue. By these simple means, I have had good success in restoring children afflicted with paralysis. You may also use a cupping process to bring the blood to the spine. With a massage cup, you will be able to aid the revitalization of the nerves that are involved; namely, those lying between the shoulder blades. Do all this for possibly three months. Then commence to give the boy arm exercises. Be sure he gets nothing but live food. Always let him choose what he likes best. Be careful not to encourage overeating, for live food is 100 per cent nourishing. If he eats too much, he may expect a headache. Let him wait until he gets really hungry.

Q. Are those children who eat uncooked food exclusively, immune from infantile paralysis?

A. Such natural food makes them immune, provided it is really natural and well-balanced; also provided other conditions of a healthy life, such as fresh air, water, exercise, and rest, are complied with.

PATENT FOODS

Q. Do you advise the use of any patent compounds if they are made up of natural foods?

A. Beware of all patent preparations. I could make many varieties of them if I cared to, but I do not. I want you, instead, to know precisely what you eat— its name, how it grows, and its value. Though the manufacturers may even tell you how they prepare their products, and the ingredients they contain, each person has a different need and may not want that particular mixture at all. Your only doctor is your taste-buds, which indicate correctly your remedy. The compounds that someone has prepared fit the needs of perhaps one person out of a hundred. Don't take the chance. Get from fresh live foods, purchased at the fruit market, all the elements you need. No boxed-up calcium, iron, or other mineral is ever as good—or as cheap.

PHILOSOPHY OF LIVE FOOD

Q. Live food is said to impart to those who eat it

power and energy which cooked food lacks. Just what is the nature of this power?

A. Where does natural food get its invincible power? One can no more answer that than one can explain electricity, and yet certain general principles are evident to all who have seen what this food can accomplish. Fruits, in general terms, are electrical in their nature, while vegetables are magnetic. Magnetic forces are able to penetrate anything, even glass and rubber, so-called non-conductors. Nothing can shut out magnetism, but electricity can be guided and forced to contain itself within limits. All the herbs, root vegetables, and tubers are magnetic, but all fruits and nuts are electrical. The peanut is magnetic, since it is not really a nut, but a nut pea, grown underground.

These electrical and magnetic forces exert unbelievable power. Some real estate men were once boasting about the great fertility of their land because a pumpkin or melon planted under a wire automobile wheel grew up into the wheel, blossomed, and bore fruit, the pressure of the expanding pumpkin or melon finally becoming so great as to twist the sturdy spokes out of shape. In order to get the pumpkin or melon out, the spokes had to be cut. It seems marvelous that the growth of an apparently weak plant could do such a Herculean task. Vegetation can cause avalanches of great rocks on mountain sides. Should a seed get into the crevice of a rock and start growing, it will expand, and keep on expanding; will force its powerful roots into the rock, aided by moisture, air, and sunshine, until at last that rock will break and slip into the depths below. That is something that perhaps a huge machine could not have brought about. Some people say: "I do not see how foods can cure my disease and rebuild my body." Of course, they will not when you cook the life out of them. They are then dead. But take them directly from Nature's hand and you will see what they can do. A cooked wheat kernel will not grow, but a grain of raw wheat will. Everything cooked is dead; scarcely any life or vito remains in it.

Q. Is it true that the higher a fruit grows the more food value it has?

A. The higher a fruit grows, the more electric its nature, and the more effective it is as an eliminator, but not as a builder. The best builders are roots and herbs, that grow in or near the earth. Fruit is wonderful food for you, mornings, to completely arouse you out of your sleep and stimulate you to action. At night eat the roots, grown in the darkness of the soil, and then your digestive organs will be ready to do the repair work of your body while you are asleep as the roots once were, in darkness. Nuts, grown also on trees, always go well with fruits, and they are a true building food. When we have once recovered from the effects of wrong living and made ourselves strong, then we may live on natural tree foods—the fruits and nuts. The "fruit of the seed-bearing tree," and tree nuts, are man's natural food, it is true, but you must get well first. Tree foods are extremely powerful, and if, in your weakened state, you should eat them exclusively, your mind might become affected. Take some vegetables noon and night, to balance the diet for the time being and keep you down to earth. When we get ourselves physically normal, healthy and strong, then we should live on fruits and nuts.

Q. Is it necessary to have faith in any doctor or health system before good results may be expected?

A. I notice the modern medical dictionary does not list the word "faith" at all. Many people, however, have come to me who seemed to believe so strongly in me and my instructions, and who went to work with such sincerity, that it seemed a pleasure for them to get well, all, apparently, because of faith in what I had told them. On the other hand, I have had patients who said: "Doctor, I have no faith in you at all, but I am coming here to satisfy my mother (or daughter, or some friend)." One of this latter type said his daughter had persuaded him to come to me. He said he was going to take only one course, and if it did good, all right, and if not, all right. I replied: "It does not matter whether you have faith in me or not, but will you do what I ask?" He said he would. There were only seven lessons in that course. They were stretched far apart and he did not come often. At the end, he said: "I feel better. I have not felt so well in a long time. My chronic headaches are gone." I told him to continue to live that way and they would not trouble him again. I had his wife and daughter back of me all the while. He got well and became one of my best supporters.

That is how we helped a man who had no faith and yet got well. I have always declared that I do not require faith. All I want is that things are done according to my instructions. True, if you have faith that certain things will help cure you, they may produce a wonderful and quick cure. Faith without works will not do; neither will prayer without works. In order to get well, you must do something to build health. For instance, you must take proper food into your system. Food replenishes worn tissues, tissues that are wearing out daily. Now, if you believe it to be a fact that when you eat dead food your live tissues cannot be replenished, you must do something in order to get an answer to your prayer. What? It may be that you have been led to think, "Why is the dumb animal never sick?" and you decide the solution is that it eats no cooked food—only fruits, nuts, etc. You next think possibly fruits would be good eating for you. Experiment brings satisfaction, and these fruits are an answer to your prayer. Fruits are active. They have the dynamic force put into them by sunshine, air, and water. The salt of the earth has been concentrated in them. When these are eaten uncooked and unspoiled, there will be new dynamic energy in your blood. The answer to your prayer will be at hand; but if you should merely pray and continue to live at the same time on the old flesh and cooked food diet, your prayers would be all in vain.

There are special kinds of food for the different organs of our body. We have a great variety of natural foods, and it was not intended that we should live permanently on just one variety. Our tastebuds, normalized, will direct us. In this way we are always kept in tune, healthy and strong; have a strong vibration, and soon become as nearly 100 per cent perfect as we can. For live food never leaves any possible thing undone. It will keep on working as long as there is something to do, to perfect. After you have cleansed your body and every organ is running normally, then this food will start to sensitize, tune up, and polish the whole system. Your sense of smell, sight, and hearing, everything will be brought into a higher vibration, so that you will be able to function almost like a radio, to practice mental telepathy, and tune in on levels now inaccessible.

What a great force there is in one person's mind! How much more there must be in the collective minds of a thousand persons, who, together, project the same thought when a cripple or sick man is healed by the prayer and faith method. This force gets that person so out of himself, the collective impact of all these minds upon him is so great, that he feels transformed, healed, at once. But faith healers usually forget to say, afterward: "Go thy way and sin no more," forget to tell the one healed precisely what to do and what not to do. Both the healer and the healed are ignorant of the true cause of the disease or malformation. Suppose the healed were told to eat live food, and helped to fulfill the prayer by deeds? Then they would really get well and stay well. You may have faith. That will help. But you must also do something, because your body is built up of material substance. Influence of so many minds will have an effect on you, but it will wear off. However, when you go to work and support it by sunshine, air, water, and natural foods, and get into harmony with Nature, then you will certainly win out, and your prayer will be permanently answered. There is spiritual food as well as physical and mental food. Physical food is derived from roots and herbs; spiritual food from the fruits. By the way, really fine spiritual food is found in the aroma of flowers—their scent is food for the brain.

To sum up, faith healing without works is not very valuable, but when you practice your faith and do something to help it along, then you may expect to have excellent results.

Q. Is not morality, rather than health, the thing in life most worth while?

A. When you live on 100 per cent natural food, you build health every day of your life. You will get a better intellect, a stronger nervous system, a more powerful body, and an excellent character, because you will be free from disease, pollution, and evil. Then, naturally and easily, comes the true beauty of life: power to love others. Nothing will build better morals, stronger character, bigger and more tender hearts, than the natural way of living.

Q. Is morality natural, or does it have to be taught?

A. If we live a natural life, one in accordance with the design of Nature, we are kept naturally moral. We cannot then do anything really immoral, no matter how hard we try. If you were to try smoking a cigar, or even sitting among others who smoke, you would have to get out or get sick. As to liquor, you will be compelled to abstain from the use of it—it would come up just as quickly as you swallowed it. A puff or two of a cigar, and you will vomit. You are clean, and when you put anything into your body that does not belong there, Nature, which is in harmony with the sun, moon, and stars, and with the food that grows on the earth, will refuse it. So with other immoral practices.

Q. Have not all the inventions and marvelous developments in this world for the last twenty-five years, been due to meat eating and to stimulating drinks?

A. Meat eating does not lead to inventive ingenuity, but to rheumatism. Every pound of meat or fish contains fourteen or more grains of uric acid. All liver contains nineteen grains of uric acid per pound, and every pound of sweetbreads seventy grains of uric acid. You eat meat and seem to be stimulated. I can tell you why. The acid whips your nerves, just as a driver whips a horse. The animal will trot a little, then slow down; trot a little more, and slow down, until he drops. That is precisely what you are doing when you eat meat—you whip your body until it drops, or you find yourself with hardening of the arteries, arthritis, apoplexy, cancer, or tuberculosis. Dr. Haig, of London, an experienced doctor, states that meat eating is the cause of nearly all disease.

Q. Is it possible for us to live healthily in a big city?

A. Any individual born in a natural environment loves sunshine, air, water, and the out-of-doors, away from the smoke, dust, and congested civilization. To be obliged to live in a large city is extremely unfortunate. There we find a concentration of evil and wickedness. There, too, is the poorest environment for health. We get in the habit of living in these places, in their rush and roar; then if we go into the country, we say: "I feel out of place because it is too lonely." We seem to want all the noise, and dust, and smoke; if we don't have it, we seem to feel there is something wrong. Many a woman has told me: "I like city life. I cannot endure it in the country." These women are unnatural. They are "denaturized" so badly that they have no desire for beauty and quietness. When men get to be fifty or thereabouts, they begin to understand that it is not good to live in congested districts. They begin to see that there is something wrong with our modern civilization, that they possibly have lived long enough in that environment to have been injured physically and mentally. One thing is sure: that living continuously in this kind of environment is not conducive to the best health. These live food dining rooms, however, even in this great city, will give you, in the foods they serve, oxygen, nitrogen, and pure hydrogen, elements you would otherwise breathe if you were in the country. There, much oxygen and nitrogen are in the air; and perhaps, on the mountain tops, or out on the ocean, we may even get a little ozone. This last is very precious. In the city ozone is absent, but in the country, especially in forests, we may detect it. Then how delicious it smells! What a difference in the city air after even a little rain! It seems as though the atmosphere were washed. Is it not too bad that the air we breathe most of the time is so polluted that a little rain can make a difference? Yet we get into the habit of living in this environment, and think nothing about it until it is firmly ingrained.

Civilization is doing things very rapidly nowadays to overcome some of these conditions. Modern improvements and equipment are being applied to bring to us better air and ventilation, even to the extent of creating artificial ozone, which, however, is not yet fine enough and correct enough to be suitable for extensive inhalation. Some doctors have instruments that make ozone, but these alone are not enough to cast off the accumulated bad conditions in the human anatomy. They alone cannot yet dissolve the phlegmy condition of the body, though some day we may succeed in getting to that stage of perfection. Then we shall have a new habit—that of breathing manufactured air, air that is more pure than that of the general city atmosphere. This may come about by a mechanical device to take the air, wash it, and add the proper oxygen, nitrogen, and ozone that we burn out with the fumes of vehicles. These fumes are responsible for reducing the volume and quality of our air. The high percentage of carbon dioxide makes city air almost impossible, but we get into the habit of inhaling it and do not think of the harm it is constantly doing us.

Our skin is not white. It is only made white by wearing clothes and being shut up behind walls. We, therefore, who live in cities and do not get the full-bodied sunshine, or fresh, pure air and water, must be dependent all the more for the maintenance of our health upon natural foods, foods which have never been cooked. In them there are stored the air, the water and the sunshine which cause the vegetables and fruits to grow. No matter whether you spend most of the time in office, store, or elsewhere in an artificial environment, you will have in natural food much stored-up health and vitality. When you eat it you will get that normal vibration which is necessary for perfect health. Remember this when you are in the city, so polluted by gasoline fumes and assorted varieties of smoke and unnatural smells.

Q. Is it possible to live on live food in a cold climate?

A. Certainly. It does not matter how cold or how warm the climate, you should always be well. If you live on natural live foods that are raised in the climate where you reside, it makes no difference whether there is summer temperature today and below zero tomorrow. I lived in the Dakotas and Minnesota where there was just such weather. It did not trouble me more than the rest. I did not wear overshoes, and would carry my overcoat on my arm. Then people would ask me how it was I could keep warm. When I would tell them I was eating nothing but raw food, they really did wonder how I could keep warm. That is all prejudice and ignorance, to be sure.

You cannot become warm by eating cooked foods. They are dead. If you eat them hot, they will develop slight temporary heat in your system, but when that is gone, you feel colder than before because the dynamic force is lacking. But when you eat live foods they will stimulate the body to create its own warmth, as well as furnishing you with natural fat and carbohydrates, which are heat-produ,ing fuels. Horserad-ish is very warming. So, too, are foods which contain oil, starch, and natural sugar. Both honey and dried fruits are excellent for a cold day. Add some olive oil and honey to a starchy food, like the banana. A half hour after eating you will feel a great deal warm-er. Sometimes, in the Dakotas, I ate raw oats, which contain a great number of heat-producing calories. Put on oil and honey, and you will feel the warmth going through the veins. That is the way to heat your body, not with clothes, and not with cooked food.

Q. Are tropical fruits good for us northerners?

A. All plants are compatible with the earth, air, and water, elements of the climate in which they grow. All the foods grown in California are for those people living in this climate. If you live in the state of Washington, Florida, or North Dakota, you should, as far as possible, eat only the products of your particu-lar section of the country.

Q. Do you think that human life can be main-tained indefinitely on raw food alone?

A. Old-fashioned people say humans cannot thrive on uncooked food. How is it that all our horses, sheep, cows, hogs, and all of our wild animals, are rarely ill and live so long? How is it that they live from six to ten times their age of maturity, whereas man lives only about two and one-half times his age of maturity? A horse, for example, is mature at three years. It often gets to be twenty-five, and sometimes thirty or more years old. Cows, which are also mature at three, live to be fifteen or twenty. Hogs mature at one year, and sometimes reach ten, or more. Man, on the other hand, is fairly well developed only at twenty. By the same ratio, he should live at least seven times that number of years, or one hundred forty. Why are we the shortest-lived animals? Because we dig our graves with our teeth, day by day, when we eat the lifeless foods which are still quite universally consumed.

Q. How long have you lived on live food?

A. About twenty years. I live very carefully because I prize that goal I hope to attain. Yet I have found, because my body was so deteriorated, that it took a great portion of these twenty years to get me purified. In the last year or two I see I am gradually obtaining a new force and a new energy. I hope I myself shall arrive at that degree of force, dynamic energy, and brilliance of intellect, that we all should have. Live right and time will bring with it all those qualities and powers we universally crave. I know that these come slowly to one who has started out on this road long after becoming a grown man. I was close to fifty before I saw the light. I recommend this system to all ages.

Q. When a person begins to eat live food, how long before a crisis appears?

A. It depends upon the condition of your body. You may expect a crisis, ordinarily, in about three months. Sometimes, however, it comes immediately. I find that it depends upon how well the individual understands himself and his own idiosyncrasies. If he hits upon the right food, the one which he likes best, at the outset, and is persistent in its use, he may get his crisis quite early, say within a week, and will commence to eliminate in earnest. Some, however, do not arrive at this point before three months, six months, or even a year or two.

Q. How long before a sick person's body will become normal with a raw food diet?

A. It will take you at least three to five years, and possibly seven, before your body is rebuilt out of live material. If you begin late, say at forty-five or fifty, it will require a still longer period. It also depends upon how faithfully you live on these foods. If you are in earnest and live strictly in accordance with your best knowledge, you will be rebuilt much more quickly than if you dabble now and then in cooked food. Another consideration in the length of time required is the condition of your body. If you have not abused it to any great extent, have not taken drugs and injections, or smoked, it will take a shorter time to become normal than if you had.

Q. How long will it be before I am immune from disease? I have just started on the live food diet.

A. It may take from six to twelve months before you arrive at a condition of immunity. In those months, Nature will be cleaning your body, getting rid of the waste matter and poisons that have been accumulating during your past life. You are going to feel anywhere from five to twenty-five years younger than before you began. You must, however, be sure always to get 100 per cent health-building material for the body forces to work with. That is what you need, not the contents of a drug store, or medical doc· tors to tell you that you must have an operation to get this or that diseased organ out of your body. Common sense and persistence always win the day.

Q. You say live food cleanses the system. Will it keep on doing that even after my body has been relieved of disease?

A. Nature, through live food, works upon the body and mind as long as there is something to be improved upon. It will keep right on perfecting your system until you have become near-perfect, and that, for most of us, means many years indeed of effort and conscientious living. Were you to discontinue the use of live food exclusively after ridding your body of disease, it would not take long before you would again become unwell. Besides, in order to function to the maximum capacity, to do your best both mentally and physically, the live food diet is essential.

Q. Is it dangerous to change from cooked food to raw food at once, or should there be a gradual tapering off? Should one satisfy a renewed craving for the old food?

A. The answer to your first question is no, start at once. Throw away all the cooking utensils; keep all spices out of your sight. Do not let anything remain about that will tempt you, anything that indicates wrong living. If you are milk hungry, make a milk out of nuts. Keep away from the odor of cooking. All this may not be essential for one who has developed a strong will-power, but it is wise to make the change as easy for oneself as possible.

You will, after living a while on the live food diet, get a strong craving for the articles of your former diet. Do not resist the temptation by suppressing it—go and prepare whatever you desire in the way of cooked food, just as you have been accustomed to making it. Have it put on the table, but (and this is important) a raw salad, too, or whatever raw food you like best. Start eating the cooked food, but only in very tiny morsels. Roll it on your tongue until thoroughly insalivated; chew it thoroughly; do not swallow before it has been reduced to a semi-liquid. When your taste has been thoroughly satisfied in this manner, finish your meal with the raw foods, and notice how much better they taste. Under no circumstances should you gulp the cooked food down in large mouthfuls—that will bring back the old cooked-food habit in full force. Cooked food, when craved, if eaten as I have directed, will act as a medicine for the perverted tastebuds, and will help normalize them. This abnormal craving will appear now and then, but at less frequent intervals as time goes on.

Q. Is seventy-one years too old to start on natural foods?

A. Years make no difference. You should not think that you are old until you are at least two hundred. No one is really old these days—we are all mere children. If you are to learn anything on this earth, you should live at least five hundred years, according to

George Bernard Shaw, and go to school every day of your life. I have known of many elderly people achieving splendid, robust health when they were afflicted by grave diseases or low vitality. One, who made the change at the age of seventy, is regaining his hearing, which had been bad for many years; has been completely cured of a long-standing case of eczema; and is able to walk five or six miles in one day, whereas formerly he puffed and panted after walking a couple of blocks. Even assuming that your body is practically worn out, you can revitalize it through the vito in uncooked foods and by proper living in other respects, such as exercise and conservation of the vital forces.

Q. Is it safe to change to the raw food diet after living on a great deal of meat?

A. Is it safe to stay in a burning building when you can walk out and save yourself? When God gives you the most natural, most delicious foods in the world, can you ask if it is safe to eat them just because they are raw and in harmony with sunshine, air, and the water of the earth? Our primitive ancestors, before the discovery of fire, lived entirely on uncooked food. Man has eaten meat only under compulsion, when other and more delicious foods were lacking. With the discovery of the use of fire, he learned to broil, bake, fry, and stew it. This increased the repertoire of flavors and made it more palatable. However, although man has eaten meat, both cooked and uncooked, for ages, our bodies have not changed sufficiently anatomically to eat animal food without harm.

Our colon, for example, is much too long for the meat to pass through before fermentation and putrefaction set in. Meat-eating animals, such as tigers, cats, and wolves, have a very short colon, which enables the meat to be passed through quickly. The teeth of human beings are similar to those of frugivorous apes, our remote ancestors, according to the scientists; incisors, or eye teeth, lack the length and sharpness necessary for the tearing of raw flesh. Moreover, the body is not equipped to handle, without ultimate damage, the excess uric acid contained in even a small quantity of meat. If we were intended by Nature to be meat eaters, we would be able to take care of the excess, but we are not. Some say their tastebuds have craved meat from the time they were children. Now, if our tastebuds crave meat and our bodies are damaged by the eating of such foods, we may reasonably conclude not that Nature intended us to eat meat, but that our tastebuds have been perverted. Perversion may, and usually does, begin at a very early age. A baby raised on cows' or goats' milk, sometimes even from birth, is in no position to judge intelligently as to its proper food on arriving at the age when it can take solid fare.

Q. Is it possible to maintain strength for strenuous work or play on live food?

A. A man who was a raw foodist once remarked to me, "I have just been on a long hike in the mountains. I walked miles, carrying a thirty-pound burden. The chap who was with me carried twenty pounds. I, as you know, am a raw fooder, but he eats meat and po-

tatoes, just as most people do. He was proud of his
hiking ability and was going to show me up and prove
that one could not do strenuous exercise without being
sustained by flesh foods. Well, he was all in before
night came." He continued by saying that he had not
only kept up with his companion, but that on the morning when he came back from the trip he had most of
his food left, enough for another hike. His companion
had to take the train home from the foot of the mountains, but our raw fooder did not—he kept on walking.
He told me he felt fine, had eaten very little, mostly
dried fruits and nuts. To look at him, one could see
he had plenty of endurance, power, and energy, together with a glance that spoke sincerity and truth.
And remember, he was only an amateur, not a profes-
sional hiker.

Another case I have in mind is this: Not long ago,
a tailor in Long Beach bought a ten-acre plot of ground
near Corona. In potato-planting time he said to the
man he had hired to help with the gardening, "I shall
come out Sunday and help with the hoeing." The gardener laughed, and replied, "You will have to eat some
beefsteak before you come. Your raw food might be
all right when tailoring, but down here on the ranch
it's different—you will have to do some beefsteak eating." "All right, I'll show you," the tailor responded.
When Sunday came, he took some apples along for his
lunch, found his hoe, and went into the garden to work.
Then came the test. The regular gardener was quite a
distance ahead of him at the start, but it did not take
long before the tailor gained on him, and before the
morning was half gone the tailor was far ahead. He

kept right on going, and when noon hour came, the other man, saying he was going to have dinner, started for the house. The tailor did not stop; he kept right on working. Before the day was up the tailor had done more than twice the work the other chap had. Finally, the gardener asked, "How do you do it?" The answer came easily to the tailor, "Eat more apples." Half seriously, the other returned, "Well, I'm going downtown soon to get a box of them."

Q. What is the cause of physical and mental tiredness?

A. Mental weariness always follows physical exhaustion. When the physical body is tired and does not seem to be able to recuperate, your mind cannot function properly either. Cooked food has little or no nourishment in it. If you eat it, you are simply starving yourself. Many seem to have the idea that no one can live continuously on raw foods. Now, raw food is live food, and cooked food is dead food, dead material. When your food is denatured, you eventually denature your whole system; you get out of harmony with the natural elements of the earth on which you live. The sunshine will seem an enemy, fresh air an enemy. In the case of a cooked-fooder, sunshine will cause sunburn, and sometimes sunstroke—all this because the sunshine, fresh air, and water are in harmony with natural food and not with the dead food he is putting into his body, and of which his tissues have been built up. When you put flesh or cooked vegetables into your stomach, you are truly burying it, as you bury other dead and decaying material in the earth.

The flesh-eating animals, such as the tiger, lion, vulture, and the like, are all far beneath man in the order of evolution. Man is the highest type of animal life, and therefore should live on the highest order of food; namely, nuts, fruits, herbs, and root vegetables. In man's perfect state he could maintain himself on fruits and nuts; that would be the proper thing to do. But in man's present state of development he must have herbs and roots. If man had never, so to speak, fallen from grace by eating dead, cooked food, he would now be on a far higher plane both physically and mentally. But instead of being perfect, he has wasted his strength through all kinds of dissipation and abuse. He cannot now subsist on the diet proper to the perfect man. In spite of his years he must begin in Nature's kindergarten. In other words, he must build up his depleted body by the use of vegetables and roots, as well as the higher types of food which will be suitable to a later stage of his development. So eat a balanced ration of fruit, herbs, and roots, all uncooked, together with a few flaked nuts. Your mental condition will then soon be cleared away. You will be able to think, to work, all day long, and in the evening you will not feel tired.

Q. Why does one get weak when starting the raw food life?

A. Because your system is full of mucous from cooked food. Your digestive organs, as yet, cannot assimilate natural foods as they should—they are clogged up. It will take from two to three weeks, at least, to clean them out, then from four to six months before your blood has gained its proper constituents. But in a year's time you will be able to hold your own with any man, and you will be immune from all disease.

Q. Are there not many people who eat cooked food and are at the same time strong and healthy?

A. Their strength comes from muscular activity, from contact with fresh air and sunshine, not from the food they eat. The food really prevents the organs from functioning to their full capacity; mucous and waste matter accumulate, forming fertile culture beds for countless disease germs. These diseases may lie latent for many years before they distress the individual noticeably. By the time a cooked fooder arrives at the age of sixty, his body is practically exhausted from its continuous battle with unnatural foods and other strength-depleting agents, and his system is ripe for a final rebellion. His whole body rises up in the form of an acute disease like pneumonia; or a chronic disease, like heart disease or cancer, may send out its ghastly signals. He attributes these diseases to old age, naturally, but it is really not old age at all. Instead, it is the inevitable result of improper diet and disobedience to natural law in general.

Live for one year on these foods and you will find your muscles becoming sinewy. After two years, you will commence to realize that you are the possessor of wonderful strength. In three years' time, you will realize that your wrinkles have departed, and after five years you will feel twenty-five years younger—not only feel it, but look it.

Q. I have been on raw foods for over a year. Why am I so weak? Sometimes I seem to have no will power.

A. This is where a little knowledge of psychology can help you. You must learn how to concentrate on the idea of power. When you go to bed tonight, put your hand over your forehead, close your eyes; then say to yourself, "I will be strong. No one shall have power over me. I will control all my physical functions, and I will not yield to any weakness." Keep your hand in position until you fall asleep. Do that every night and your negative state will be transformed into a positive one. Natural physical stimulation will help you also. Every morning, after rising, take a cold shower bath, rub down dry, and do your daily dozen with a vim. Keep on, and you will certainly get strong in the end.

Q. Why are women weaker than men? Is it natural? I have read stories about the ancient Amazons, each of whom was a match for a dozen men.

A. A girl I know, nineteen years old, who has never eaten anything cooked, nor dairy products, has proved herself equal in contest to any two average men. Her father said that once he hired two men to load up a truck with honey and take it to market. The honey was packed two sixty-pound cans in a case. That meant one hundred twenty pounds per case, plus the weight of the cans and the box, which amounted to about ten or fifteen pounds. The two men talked the matter over and decided one was to take hold of one end of the cases, the other of the other end, and hoist them up in that fashion. When this girl saw how they were putting the boxes onto the truck, she walked up and asked, "Can't one of you put these cases up and the other arrange them in place?" One said, "I suppose we could, but it is easier this way." Then she replied, "You both get up and I'll keep you busy." And she did. The two of them had all they could do to get the cases stacked away. This was done by the nineteen year old raw food girl. I say it again, the strongest people on earth are those who live entirely on natural food. Women can develop their muscles as well as men.

Q. Please tell us why living on natural foods keeps one thin.

A. Natural food does not keep you "thin," but normally proportioned. It will never produce adipose tissue. That is because there is plenty of adhesive tissue present in it. Adhesive tissue never allows you to become corpulent. Many people who do not eat live food are really thin, because they are starved for want of genuine nourishment. What I have said of live foods refers to individuals who have already rebuilt their body tissues and bones on live food. Before this has been accomplished, however, the half-dead material of which your body is composed must be eliminated, gradually, it is true, but none the less certainly, under the cleansing influence of the true food dynamic. Naturally, your friends will tell you that you look half starved, that your bones project, when in truth it is they who are starved, though they may appear to be well fed. Give yourself time, and you will build a beautiful, graceful body.

Q. If live food is more nourishing than cooked food, why is it that you can keep fleshier on cooked food than on live food?

A. Cooked food creates adipose tissue, which means that the cells are enlarged and in a bloated condition, forming, thereby, genuine storehouses for waste matter. Regardless of what your friends or relatives may think, this bloated tissue is not a sign of health. It is not firm tissue or normal tissue; it does not indicate strength or vitality.

Q. Is it a fact that one can abuse raw food by too complex mixing and overeating?

A. Live food will not do you any real harm in whatever quantity or mixture you eat it, provided always your tastebuds have sought it out and your stom-ach does not rebel. Always judge by results. However, if raw food will take away the desire to smoke, it will also gradually eliminate the desire for overeating, as well as for complicated mixtures. I have known two or three people who were tremendously big eaters of raw food. That was during the days when their bodies were being built up to normal. They were not satisfied at any meal unless they had two or three plate-fuls, and they kept this up, one for two years and the other for two and one-half. Then something happened —a crisis, or acute elimination, set in. The body had stored up enough energy to once and for all make a thorough sweep of the poisons in the system. At the time of this crisis, they stopped eating—in fact, did not touch any food for from three to six weeks. They seemed to feel much over-nourished; they could not look at food. When they resumed eating, they ate al-most as little birds, scarcely enough, one thought, to keep them alive. Yet each of them does vigorous manual work—one is a painter, who eats only once a day, and then only very little.

Q. Do you recommend eating the same kind of fruits every day for any length of time?

A. The tastebuds know what you want and need. When your "master builders" get signals from your body that a certain kind of food has become unnecessary and that another kind of food is desired instead, they will indicate it clearly and quickly. Therefore, be guided by them rather than by any cut and dried system of diet, or advice from others who may be well-meaning but ignorant as to what your body requires.

Q. Is it not more natural to eat fruit than herbs? It seems to taste better.

A. Yes. Fruit is man's natural food. However, we, in our abnormal state, after having lived on flesh food and cooked material for so many years, require the herbs and roots for the rebuilding of our bodies to a state of normalcy, since these are richer in mineral salts than fruits. We must live on a balanced diet of fruits, nuts, herbs, and roots for quite some time before our bodies are readjusted to the higher vibration of the fruitarian diet. We must assimilate as much rich earth salts as we possibly can so that our bodies will be built up quickly and sturdily. Your taste will change as your body develops. At first, you may have a craving for cabbage or for oranges. Later on, you may crave tomatoes, or avocados, or grapefruit.

It is well for you to sample as many different types of fruits and vegetables as are on the market. You may find that you like certain types of vegetables in their natural form very well indeed. On the other hand, you may be eating vegetables in salads which your taste-buds would rebel against if eaten alone. For instance, you may never have eaten uncooked cauliflower or asparagus, or uncooked turnips or rutabagas, yet these may appeal to you and be just what you need. If you have a craving for a bitter food, such as sun-dried olives or the various wild herbs, you should eat them. Avocado rinds, chewed or eaten with the inside, will give you much of this same bitter element, and further-more are delicious when eaten in combination with the oily so-called "flesh." The rind of the thin-skinned varieties, such as the Fuerte and the small late summer "seedlings," should by all means be eaten with the rest of the avocado. Some of the darker-skinned varieties contain so much of this bitter element that you may not be able to eat a great deal of it. These rough rinds, when swallowed, will act as good sweeping material for your bowels, also.

Q. Is there any herb, fruit, or leaf naturally poison-ous to the human body?

A. No. However, you must remember that any-thing you eat because of some reason other than that you like it, or seem to crave it, will do you harm and will in that sense be a poison. If you are not sure whether a thing is of value to you, try a tiny bit of it. If you feel no ill effects, try a little more next time, and so on. It is always wise to do this in the case of fruits, vegetables, or plants with which you are not familiar. It is well to experiment, but take precautions as to quantity. Our Creator did not give us food in order to kill us, but rather that we might live long on this earth and be happy, full of health and vitality. Surely, we can trust that He has created food which is perfect in the natural state, food that we could not improve on.

Q. Is it true that live fooders, if hurt, will never carry a scar?

A. Live fooders' wounds heal without a scar. This is not so of those who eat cooked food, for their blood is not right. When a wound or operation leaves a scar, we know at once that the patient has been living on cooked food. Why? Because there is nothing in cooked food, or the blood derived therefrom, that will replace in a natural way injured tissue or bone. Scar tissue is only phlegmy material which has, so to speak, been thrown into the breach in the absence of true tissue-building substance. Natural food does not allow scar tissue to be formed. Blood built up on live food will replace every worn-out or injured cell in your body as the need arises.

Q. Is it not true that farm animals do well on cooked food? Farmers usually boil the potatoes which they feed their hogs.

A. Fat hogs are contrary to Nature. Only lean hogs could survive the rigor of a natural existence. But what the farmer desires is plenty of poundage so as to make a real impression on the scales—and purse—of the buyer when they are sold. Wild animals, however, as well as cows and horses, do not habitually eat cooked food as we do.

Once a man who was very ill came to see me. He told me about his herd of fine cattle. They had gotten sick; so he fed them on boiled potatoes. Instead of getting well, they got worse. The first thing he knew, they were dying, and he was losing big money, because they were high-bred cattle and every one dead meant a loss of a couple of thousand dollars. He lost six of the herd. Some time after that, he himself became sick, and it was then that he came to see me. I explained to him the importance of diet, that he must not eat anything cooked. Astonished, he asked, "Nothing cooked at all?" "No," I replied, "nothing cooked." "How about raw potatoes?" he asked. I told him that if he liked them, they were all right. Then he said, "Perhaps those cooked potatoes were the reason my cows died." His reasoning was correct. He was very careful after that to see that the cattle and horses got the very cleanest raw foods, nothing cooked. Farmers usually give cattle, horses, and chickens the best food, and themselves the poorest. We, like the animals, require vital raw foods in order to be healthy and happy. Why not give ourselves a chance?

Q. How is it that people are able to sustain life on cooked food?

A. If we observe carefully the diet of the average individual, we will find that he eats a fair percentage of uncooked food in one form or another, as for instance apples, oranges, grapes, and other fruits, as well as green vegetables. A very little real food, apparently, can go a long way, if necessary. In addition to this, we have the beneficent influence of sunshine and fresh air, physical exercise, water, and rest. Many cooked food·ers, in these latter respects, lead a rather wholesome life.

All so-called vitamines, A, B, C, etc., are really not vitamines at all, but alkalis. True, some of these remain in the food after it has been cooked, but the true life, or vito, has been totally lost by the high temperature to which the food has been subjected. Certain forms of life, as for instance the Mediterranean fruit fly, can be destroyed by a temperature of not much above that of the human body—112° F. Food vito is no doubt a very sensitive form of life also, and we shall do well to protect it from all unnatural conditions previous to the food's appearance on the table. While the life-giving elements are not to be found in cooked food itself, during the process of cooking the vito escapes in the form of invisible particles susceptible only to the nos·trils. It is the application of heat, not the particular method or device used, that does the damage; pressure cookers, fireless ovens, slow, quick, or medium heat with or without water, make no difference.

Q. Should persons of different chemical types eat the same kind of food?

A. Every individual has an idiosyncrasy of his own, regardless of type. All should select their food according to the tastebuds, our master builders. Whatever natural food the master builders indicate a desire for, we should eat. Whatever chemical element is most in demand will be selected by our body according to need. Some foods contain more of a certain element, say, iron, or sulphur, than do others. You need not necessarily eat the food that is richest in the particular element your body needs, since all foods contain at least a small amount of practically every one of the sixteen elements. You may, however, have to eat more food than you would if ate that in which the necessary element or elements are concentrated. Always depend upon your tastebuds—it simplifies life.

Q. Would it not be advisable to have a medical doctor diagnose one's case before undergoing any kind of treatment?

A. By their own record, the physical diagnoses of the medical doctors are only five per cent correct. This is stated in their own American Medical Association magazine. A doctor had investigated for over a year the correctness or incorrectness of general medical diagnosis; that is, physical diagnosis, and found that in all the hospitals in the city of New York it averaged only five per cent correct. What, therefore, would be the value of such an examination? Why not forget medical diagnosis and go to a naturopath for treatment? After all, what you want is to get rid of your ailment, whatever it may be. The basis of naturopathy is Natural Law. The naturopath teaches you how to live in accordance with Natural Law, and then you will cure yourself.

Q. Do you ever prescribe medicine?

A. Conventional medicines are poisons. They are inorganic, and the body will not absorb them. Furthermore, dead material of that kind cannot, under any circumstances, produce life and health. Rather, it is an irritant for which your blood has absolutely no use. Your blood is, or should be, alive, and it wants help when sickness comes. The blood is the principal defender of the body against all external or internal forces or materials that would destroy it. If you wish to do something to help the blood in its role as defender, you must furnish vito, which is found only in undenatured and unrefined products, uncooked. Vito harmonizes with the normal action of your blood. That kind of food is your best medicine. If congenial with your own personal taste, it has the power to restore you to health and normality.

Q. What should a live-fooder do when he gets an elimination crisis?

A. Continue on the particular food that seems to have brought out the poison, slowing down somewhat, however, and stopping it entirely for some time when you feel that the poison has been pretty well drained out. Do not be alarmed. Nature will persist in the cleansing process only as long as it is necessary.

Q. I believe in and live the raw food life, but my husband does not. Our children eat as he does. How best can I win my family over to the natural system?

A. Be a shining example of what natural living can accomplish, and you need not do any talking. Deeds speak louder than words. On the other hand, if you are not in much better condition than you were a year ago, they rightfully will not feel impressed. This situation is fruitful ground for marital disharmony. You may be able to win over your husband gradually by including in his menu tasty salads, vegetables, and fruits, in place of heavy pastries, meats, and the like. The children will find themselves thriving on uncooked fruits and salads, able to make better grades at school, as well as to outdo their companions in play.

Q. Is raw starch (potato, corn, and wheat) as digestible as cooked starch?

A. Nothing, as a rule, ferments more easily and copiously, in the stomach and intestines, than cooked starch. Nothing is more acid forming. Raw starch, on the other hand, although it may also be subject to fermentation, is alkaline in its reaction, and helps neutralize any acid already in the system. Furthermore, whereas cooked starch ferment is sour, raw starch ferment is sweet, and therefore less objectionable. If your tastebuds call for potato, corn, or any other natural unprocessed starch, do not be afraid to follow their signal.

Q. When one's stomach rebels with every meal of natural food, and it seems feverish and irritated, is it not wiser to eat steamed or baked vegetables if one cannot afford to fast or go on juices because of a weakened physical condition?

A. No one is ever too weak to go on an alternate-day fast; that is, fasting one day and eating on the next. This is the best method for bringing back strength, strength of the body, and of the stomach in particular. Whenever your stomach is highly irritable, you should not eat complex mixtures heavily seasoned. Simple, soft fruits and vegetables are the best. You cannot get strength from denatured, dead food. That is manifestly impossible; you cannot make bricks without straw.

PHLEGM

Q. What causes a sharp pain in the lungs when getting up in the morning? It is not tuberculosis, doctors tell me.

A. Your lung cells appear to be in a catarrhal condition. A very heavy phlegm has gotten into them. When these cells close up while you are asleep, the gluey phlegm, coming in contact with the opposite walls, pulls them together. Then, when you wake up in the morning and start to fill your lungs with air, you will suffer a stitch like a pin prick, or the cutting of a knife, because the breath, in refilling these cells, will tear them slightly.

To cure this, first of all put a poultice of hot onions over the chest, and keep it there all night. Lie on your back as much as possible so as to keep the poultice in place. In the morning, you will find that this phlegm has been rather well liquefied, and you will be able to expel it in large quantities. Then do the following breathing exercises: inhale until you feel the "stitch" coming back. It will not be nearly as bad as before, although bad enough. When you feel the hurt, hold your breath a moment, until it stops. Then continue the same inhalation. When it hurts again, hold, and the pain will soon go. When it lets up, draw some more air, and perhaps by that time you will hear a little "pop" down in the lung region, which means you have done what you set out to do. Hold the breath a moment, then, so that the air will make the cells moist all around, finally expelling. In this way, you save the day for your lung cells and give the phlegm a chance to be thrown out.

As soon as you have loosened some of those constricted cells, lie face down over a cot, couch or bed. Let your head hang down. Encourage coughing to get the phlegm out. When you have done this, gargle the throat with some warm, lemonized water. Then put hot and cold applications over the chest. Rub dry, and drink a glass of hot lemonade. In the morning, eat such fruits as you like best; at noon, your favorite herbs; and roots in the evening—all these, however, only in moderate quantities. Do not eat until you feel satisfied— eat only until you are very nearly satisfied, and then stop. Make it easy for your stomach. These lung pains at rising may indicate tuberculosis in its early stage, or the less serious disease of hay fever.

Q. I am troubled with phlegm in my nostrils. How can I get rid of it?

A. Add lemon juice to a little water and sniff it up the nose. Use all the lemon juice you want. It will bring results. The cause of phlegm is always wrong living, especially wrong eating. Meat, starch, and dairy products are the chief offenders in the average person's dietary.

Q. Although I have been a live-fooder for several years, I am still forced to cough up phlegm at intervals. I have no tonsils. What causes the condition?

A. You are still eliminating the poisons accumulated in previous years, before beginning the new life. This assumes that you are at the present time living a regular, wholesome life. Check up on your daily régime, particularly on your diet, and see if you can locate anything amiss. You may be eating too heavily of eliminative foods.

PILES (HEMORRHOIDS)

Q. What can be done for a bad case of bleeding hemorrhoids?

A. Bleeding piles are caused by constipation, and this, in turn, by cooked foods, dead foods that take away the power of peristalsis, or rhythmic action, from the bowels, until they become so weak, finally, that they cannot do their work. In many instances, only the fermentation of cooked food causes bowel movements once a day, sometimes only once in two, three, or four days. Normally, there should be a bowel movement after every meal.

Hemorrhoids are often from one-half to three-quarters of an inch long, and usually, then, very painful and irritative. These are simply distended veins caused by constipation, the veinous tissues and vein tubes having become weak because of poor quality of blood. Some piles at first, however, are little boils, which then break open and begin bleeding. When tissues are weak, they bleed very easily.

How can piles be cured? By curing your constipation. When the hard feces are not constantly working down into the rectum there will be no more blood congestion in that region, barring serious degeneration of the tissues. Eat laxative foods—figs are extremely good for this condition. Do this and you will be surprised to see how easily piles will disappear without recourse to the surgeon's knife. But in the process of cure they will cause you a great deal of pain at times. For this, get a fountain syringe, put in one cup of lukewarm water, and inject into the lower bowel. Let it run very slowly. Warm water will wash the tissues clean. Immediately after, insert into the rectum a little glycerine with tannin, or some olive oil. This procedure will take the pain away.

Q. Can hemorrhoids be cured without operation, and should enemas be used?

A. People suffering from hemorrhoids should be on a strict diet for some time before commencing more direct treatment. By diet I mean living on natural foods. In the morning eat fruit, at noon the leafy herbs you like best, and in the evening the roots. Follow this up for at least six months. It will get your blood in condition to do a good job when you get ready to bring it to the affected parts. In the meantime, wash out the colon with about a cupful of warm water after each evacuation, and possibly two or three times a day besides. An enema is not a cure; just an aid to keep the colon clean, to prevent putrefaction of the lower rectum.

Hemorrhoids are the product of constipation. Constipation comes from the eating of dead, cooked food, unclean, unnourishing, and a disease builder. Now, only uncooked foods that have life in them will build up blood rich in necessary hemoglobin, that will build up these troubled centers. In about six months' time, your blood will commence to get into fairly good shape. Then start taking sitz baths, followed by the use of some natural ointment. After the bath and ointment application, do these exercises: lie on your back, grasp the bed or couch on each side, swing your legs sideways, up and down, and rotate them—three movements. Do each of them several times. You thus force the muscles to absorb the blood you brought into the region by the hot water sitz bath. Finish with a warm enema. It will probably take from three to five years before you are cured; so keep right at it. The bones will have to be completely rebuilt.

Q. Can hemorrhoids be cured by diet alone or is local treatment necessary?

A. It depends on the seriousness of the hemorrhoids. If you have a simple case of hemorrhoids, where they merely protrude, you may help yourself a great deal by just eating foods which will bring the bowels into a laxative condition. Eat plenty of bulk. Never eat cooked foods, for the cause of hemorrhoids is weakened tissue. Cooked foods are dead: the sunshine, water, and air that were put into them while they were growing have been cooked out. Therefore they have no food value. They starve and weaken the tissues, paving the way for disease.

PIN WORMS

Q. Will worms cause a child to sweat at night?

A. Pin worms will annoy a child, make it very restless, cause it to pick its nose, etc. There may also be an indication of feverishness and perspiration, but that would be largely due to the child's taking a great deal of moisture in food or drink before going to bed. Night perspiration often comes from a superabundance of water in the body. We must remember that fever and perspiration are eliminative activities of the body, that, when not too prolonged or severe, are beneficial. Uncooked food will put the worms to rout.

Q. What causes a child to grit its teeth while asleep?

A. Examine the stool. You will find that there are worms present—pin worms, very likely, that aggravate the anus. A child with clean bowels will never suffer from worms. It should be fed raw foods, not cooked material, which, under certain conditions, inevitably breeds worms. I have saved a boy's life by helping him eliminate millions of worms. The doctors had given him four days to live, but after a couple of months under my treatment he was as healthy and happy as any youngster of his age. The boy had an abdomen that looked like a basket-ball, and the slime we took from it was terrible to see. He had a large lump on one side, too, which the doctors supposed was cancer. That also disappeared.

PNEUMONIA AND CONGESTION
OF THE LUNGS

Q. Do you advise the use of the poultice for lung congestion or inflammation?

A. Yes. Boil some onions; mash them; and put into a bag while hot. Press the bag down over the chest and upper ribs and leave it there all night. In the morning, it will be surprising how you will spit up phlegm that has been loosened, and the inflammation will be considerably reduced. Thus you get rid of the waste matter that has accumulated there through periods of cooked-food eating.

When a person with pneumonia feels hungry, he should eat the natural foods he likes best—fruits until twelve noon, then herbs, and in the evening roots. Also, when he is able to, he should take sunbaths between the hours of nine and eleven-thirty every morning. The sunbathing should be combined with exercise of a mild nature—say walking, or even moving the members of the body frequently while sitting in a chair. Fresh air and sunshine do their part to help liquefy the phlegm in the chest. The important point is to reduce the inflammation and to get rid of this phlegm. When this is accomplished, the patient will be well again.

Q. Is it ever necessary to puncture the lungs in pneumonia cases to get out excess liquids?

A. Such a procedure is the last resort of the medical profession, ignorant of the true cause and cure of disease, pneumonia included. Any excess liquids in the inflamed organ will be drained off by Nature herself when she is ready to do so. Give her every opportunity, and keep your money in the bank.

POISON IVY AND POISON OAK

Q. Please tell us the best remedy for poison ivy infection.

A. One very efficient remedy is this: put two pounds of baking soda in a bathtubful of warm water. You may use, instead, cream of tartar or borax. Stay in the bath for an hour, or until the swelling has gone down. If the first bath does not help you, take another after an interval of an hour or two. Wipe yourself dry and get into bed. In the morning, you will be all right. This is very good, but why should we suffer from ivy poisoning at all? A real live fooder could rub his hands and face with poison ivy or poison oak without suffering the slightest inconvenience. On the other hand, people who live on cooked food and whose bodies are saturated with cooked acids, suffer terribly at a mere touch, or even close proximity to the plants. Therefore, the true remedy is the longer, but absolutely fundamental, reform in habits of living, especially eating.

POTENCY

Q. Can virility of an elderly person be restored?

A. The eating of salt is one of the most active causes of impotency. The eating of salt, to be sure, is usually coupled with meat eating and cookery in general, all of which add their bit to the devitalizing process. Natural food, on the other hand, creates within you a dynamic force, in other words, fertility. This force is absolutely essential for your health and vigor, your ability to hold your own in the affairs of mankind.

The vital fluids are, by means of the bloodstream, transfused throughout the entire body, vitalizing and vivifying all the faculties. Concentrated, and used for a special purpose, we call it "sex fluid." The fact, however, that these two purposes are both served by the same material substance, is important and should be constantly kept in mind. Therefore, it is most necessary to conserve, and never waste, these energies.

Have you ever heard of a sterile wild animal? Why not? Because these creatures invariably live on foods that are not cooked. They do not know the destroyer, fire, but eat their grains, roots, leaves, herbs, roots, nuts, even flesh, just as they come from the hand of Nature. Where can you see anything more beautiful than the peacock or the pheasant, with tail outspread in the sunshine? Where is there anything more active and agile than the little faun, its eyes shining, its slender legs so fleet, and its coat as smooth as though it had been polished every day? How could man improve on the gracefulness of the squirrel? No artist could conceive of anything more beautiful. Observe the animals. They have no doctors, hospitals, sanitariums, or midwives, and yet they do not seem to miss such things. Beauty and gracefulness and strength are the invariable result of right eating and right living in general, be it animal or be it man.

Q. Can you recommend any natural foods particularly valuable in restoring potency?

A. Ripe avocados are fine; also tomatoes, watercress, and sun-dried black olives.

Q. What causes man to be impotent, even early in life?

A. Wild creatures remain virile until death. To be sure, those in zoos are often exceptions to this rule, for the simple reason that they have lost contact with their natural environment and habits. Man, too, has done exactly that, and his potency will return with his return to Nature and her laws. Specifically, wastage of sex energy in youth, through masturbation or sex relationships, is one of the greatest causes of later impotence.

PREGNANCY AND CHILD BIRTH

Q. Is it necessary for a woman to be under a doctor's care during pregnancy?

A. That depends upon how much she knows about herself. If she does not know how to take care of her body, it would be well to take the instructions of a good naturopath or those of a midwife, or anyone who has had experience along those lines. Exercise should not be shunned—just the reverse. Good development of the abdominal region is necessary for easy delivery. Fresh air and sunshine are always important, and especially the one hundred per cent live food diet. The expectant mother should have plenty of rest, particularly during the last months. If these directions are followed, there should be no "morning sickness," or nauseousness; neither should there be spells of dizziness.

Q. Can a woman forty-three years of age undertake to have another baby? She has two children, one twelve and one fifteen years old.

A. Every "normal" woman who has lived on natural food one hundred per cent for more than two years will be able to give birth to a child, and that painlessly. Many mothers do not, however, appreciate the necessity of living one hundred per cent on natural food, and think they can eat bread or drink milk in addition. There is real danger in that, for the organs must be supple and strong. This is impossible when the phlegm supply in the body is being constantly renewed by eating even small quantities of phlegm-producing foods. Age has comparatively little to do with capacity for or ease of birth—the principal factor is the condition of the woman's body.

Q. Would you advise any particular diet for a pregnant woman? Suppose she craves something besides fruits and vegetables that are uncooked?

A. While a woman is pregnant she should have her cravings gratified. That is one time we should be obedient to her cravings, whether they are perverted or not. She must not keep that false appetite, so root it out or it will be transmitted to her offspring. I have had a case where a woman asked for sausages; another where gin was called for, and though I object to this kind of "food," I furnished the one woman with sausages and the other with gin. Both had good results.

To relate another instance: the child in question was ten days old, would not take milk, and was commencing to die. The parents could not find out what was wrong.

An expensive medical doctor was called, but he did not seem to be able to put his finger on the trouble. I was recommended by one of my patients. When I arrived, the mother was dressed in a cream-colored silk gown, with a pearl necklace extending to the floor—actually long enough that she had to hold it up so as not to step on it. Every time she stirred this wrapper crackled like paper, and yet that poor baby would not take its milk. I looked at the baby—it was growing blue. The nurses gathered around me, as well as some of the maids. I said to the mother, "I shall have to come to you for the key to the problem." She replied, "Yes, doctor. I will do what I can to help." Then I asked her if she had had any craving during pregnancy that she did not gratify. After some thought, she said there was nothing. Immediately, one of the nurses spoke up, "Why, yes, ma'am, you remember you wanted an apple that stormy night. You would not let us go after it, and the next morning you did not want it any more." I said, "That is sufficient. Have the nurse take the child to the kitchen and feed it some freshly scraped apple." The nurse did this, and the baby started eating the apple ravenously. The nurse screamed for joy, crying in to the mother, "Oh, the baby is eating some apple." In this manner, the child's life was saved. I saw the boy two years later, and I never saw a child who looked healthier than he. So, if there be anything that a woman in a pregnant condition craves, particularly if it be a fruit or a vegetable in its natural condition, see that she gets it.

Q. Is there any difference at birth between the

babies of mothers living on uncooked foods and those living on cooked foods?

A. Certainly. The live food mother will have a smaller child, as a rule, thus making for easier delivery. This child will also be born clean, without any necessity for being bathed on its entrance into the world.

PRENATAL INFLUENCE

Q. Is it true that the character of an unborn child can be influenced by special modes of life on the mother's part, such as by alternating music, art, and science?

A. The environment of a woman in a pregnant condition should always be according to her own plan, not someone else's. Perhaps she may express a desire to live on the hillside, or out in the country, or by the lake. She may want to go into a cave. It makes no difference what she wants—her surroundings should be adjusted to her own ideas, her own desires. Also there should be no artificial program adhered to which has been arranged by others. She should consult her own deepest instincts and desires and let them guide her activities.

PROLAPSED ORGANS

Q. What would you recommend for a weak prolapsed stomach and transverse colon? I have eaten raw food for two years.

A. It is not always a certain kind of food that gets you well, but also the way in which you eat it. In the case of a prolapsed stomach, you must, as it were, force the stomach to get down to business. If you have a stomach that is about twice as large as it should be, it is lazy, inactive, has no peristaltic movement, acts only as a receptacle for food. Have your stomach work on small quantities. For instance, take about three ounces of fruit in the morning. You will soon be hungry again, but that is all right. In two or three hours, eat three more ounces. In time you will, by so doing, force that big stomach to become small. As it gets smaller it will need less room, and the organs that were previously crowded will commence to raise it up.

In the privacy of your room you should make a practice of going bear fashion, on hands and feet. Since your legs are longer than your arms, the stomach will be tilted forward. This will help your organs to get into and stay in a normal position. We do well, sometimes, to imitate the dumb animal who walks on all fours. Do this about one-half hour at a time if you can.

Remember to eat only a little every three hours: fruit before noon; herbs during the day; and one root meal, always at night. After a while, you will perhaps care for only two meals a day. Eat only just as much as you think the stomach requires. You may need to eat only one meal a day, unless you are a very hard-working individual.

Q. What causes a fallen stomach?

A. Gluttony. Many persons unconsciously seek to get certain necessary food elements by eating a great deal, rather than by following their instinct for natural food. Quality, instead of quantity, is what we want. Cooked food does not fill the bill—the stomach wants live food, with its vitality, nourishment, and pleasing taste. Even after shifting to a live food diet we may find the old habit of gluttony (really starvation) still with us for a time. It is important to eat slowly and chew your food well. If necessary, limit your food intake severely until your stomach becomes accustomed to the lesser quantity.

Q. Will a good abdominal support relieve or cure a severe case of prolapsed stomach or ascending colon?

A. No. You had better throw away the support and commence eating less. Eat in small quantities, say three ounces at a time. The reason you have a prolapsed stomach is because you were a glutton and packed your stomach until it prolapsed in all directions. Now why is it that people become gluttons? Because the system is calling for something it does not get. Yet these stupid people will keep on eating the same material all the time instead of finding out what the tastebuds really want. If you were a dumb animal you would know what you wanted. Instead, you eat just what is set before you, which is wrong. If you do not like something, do not eat it, and do not force a child or anyone else to eat what he or she does not like. Any mother or father who whips a child because it will not eat what it does not like, is worse than a brute. It is much better to let that child alone, to let it choose its own food.

Q. Can a prolapsed colon be cured?

A. It can be cured, but you must first put it back into the place where it belongs. If it is out of place by having dropped over to the side, instead of filling your stomach full and constantly pressing the colon downward and outward, eat often and in small quantities, take one-fourth as much food as you are accustomed to eat, and eat every three hours instead of every five hours. That will mean from four to six meals a day. Eating in small quantities will force this large stomach to work on small amounts. The organ will then be obliged to become smaller in order to knead the food. Being made to handle only a small intake, it will do a good job.

When your stomach has once become smaller, it will not be difficult for you to pull up that colon. Each morning, press it up into place and put a bandage over it to keep it there. Also, breathe in the following manner for a few minutes: place the hands over the colon and exhale; then pull up on the hands, leaving the colon in the proper position. Another beneficial exercise is to lie on the back and raise your feet straight up a number of times. That will strengthen the abdominal muscles. Standing on your head, or walking bear fashion, on all fours, will accomplish the same end. You should do these exercises morning and evening.

Q. Can a prolapsed uterus and bladder be corrected by eating raw food?

A. Yes. You will have to do considerable exercising, produce hyperemia (super-abundance of blood) in the affected parts, as well as restore your blood to a high degree of potency by the eating of uncooked food. The

right blood, created from the right food, is the foundation of all healing, but the other measures are valuable, sometimes necessary. Hyperemia causes contrac-
tion to take place so as to bring the organ back to its
normal position. Correct food makes your muscles
more elastic, and so it is also with a prolapsed stomach,
bladder, or uterus. First, live on natural foods for six
months so as to give your blood a chance to build up
to its proper potency. Then take a hot sitz bath, followed by a quick cold rub all over. Next walk on all
fours for some minutes. That brings your hips up high
and your chest and head low, thereby forcing all the
unnaturally sunken organs into their proper place.
This walking about bear fashion will cause the muscles
to absorb the blood you have brought there by the
hyperemia. Walk in this way as long as possible. Perhaps you may be able to do only three minutes of it at
first; later on you may be able to increase the time to
fifteen or more minutes.

PROSTATE GLAND

Q. Will you please state a remedy for an inflamed
enlarged prostate gland?

A. An enlarged prostate! It is too bad that a man
should be in this condition; but how can he help himself when he lives as most of us do—on cooked foods
that gradually paralyze all the organs? The first thing
to do is to clean out all constipation waste. You will
have to take some enemas, very likely.

Then, you should take a hot sitz-bath every night for
half an hour—a progressive heat sitz-bath. Sit in the

tub and start the water until it gets as high as the hips. Keep your legs up against the side of the bathtub and your feet up out of the water. Increase the temperature of this water until it gets to the point of endurance, and keep it there for the entire bathing period. When you get out, give your hips a cool sponging with cold water. That will close the pores of the skin and retain the heat. Immediately afterwards, lie on your back on the floor or bed and do some pelvic exercises. Bring your feet up and down and move your hips to and fro and around so as to cause the muscles there to absorb the blood attracted by the sitz-bath.

You must also eat properly, meaning uncooked fresh fruits, herbs, and roots; also nuts. Particularly should you eat the greens that act directly on the prostate. They are: mustard greens, nasturtium, and watercress —any one of them, mixed with an equal amount of lettuce.

PTOMAINE POISONING

Q. Is it possible to get ptomaine poisoning from uncooked fruits or vegetables?

A. I have known cases where people got ptomaine poisoning from watermelon which had been in the ice box with some meat. Several were sick for a week, and dangerously. I had several of these cases, all of whom recovered so quickly that they went to work next day. In short, I had caused them to get rid of the poison by giving them flour water to drink. That is the best emetic in cases of poisoning.

Excepting cases of contact or near contact with meat or cookery of all kinds, ptomaine poisoning from fruits and vegetables is unknown. Watermelon will ferment and decay, but your tastebuds will give you plenty of warning not to eat it when in that state. Even if you do eat a little, you will not be poisoned; your stomach may be a trifle sour afterwards. That is all. This is one of the most splendid things about living a natural life— that you need never worry about getting ptomaine poisoning, nor for that matter, any other kind of poisoning, provided you use reasonable care to select fruits and vegetables that have not been sprayed, sulphured, or otherwise treated by injurious chemicals. In these latter cases, even if you should happen to eat, accidentally, some injurious chemical along with the food itself, the active neutralizing and protecting agents in the uncooked fruit or vegetable would immediately set to work to segregate and eliminate it, and you would suffer little inconvenience or real damage.

Q. What is the best emergency treatment for ptomaine poisoning?

A. Ptomaine poisoning is generally caused by canned meats and sea foods that have become infected by bacteria. Occasionally, too, canned fruits and vegetables are the source of trouble, possibly due to the method used in soldering the cans. As first aid, prepare at once some flour water. Mix the flour gradually with water; stir until it becomes doughy; then dissolve the preparation with water until it reaches the consistency of milk. Give the patient one glass after another of this flour water until he has taken a quart and a half or two quarts. Then he will vomit, cleaning the stomach out thoroughly. The pressure induced by the quantity taken, lines the walls of the stomach with a sticky substance and prevents the poisonous food from affecting the membrane. The stomach will then force out all toxic matter.

If the ptomaine poisoning has been acute, you should also resort to enemas. Fill the bowels full of flour water just as you did the stomach, and when they will not hold any more let it run out. Keep on until the flour water comes out clean and there is no more odor. If, after all this, there should still be a little fever, try these vasomotor exercises: put the thumb and finger on the occipital bone. Press up against it, and forward. You will then be pressing the vasomotor nerves. These nerves connect with all the vascular organs in the digestive tract. Do this until you feel moisture on the patient's forehead, which means that you have broken the fever. Now release the inhibiting action by rotating with your fingers on each side of the bone, working upward and outward when you come near the occipital. Then give the patient these neck movements: turn the head gently back (bring it around so that it will almost touch the shoulder) and give a mild vibration; then turn the head forward again and tip it back; then turn the head over to the other shoulder, and give a vibration as before. Repeat several times.

PYORRHEA

Q. Is pyorrhea curable? What about dental preparations claiming to benefit or cure pyorrhea?

A. With the aid of live food, you can cure any disease. Pyorrhea is the accumulation of uric acid wastes in the gums. Live food will neutralize and eliminate these poisons in time. Pyorrhea is often a stubborn disease, requiring a great deal of patience in the treatment. You cannot nibble a little at cooked food now and then and expect to get rid of it.

All pyorrhea preparations are astringents, almost universally of a chemical nature, and extremely dangerous for that reason. You cannot afford to fill up your system with non-assimilable chemicals, even if the results were all that is claimed. As a matter of fact, they are not. Temporary relief is often obtained; the patient is in high glee over what appears to be his relief from suffering; but as soon as the paralyzing effect has worn off, pyorrhea is back, as bloody and irritating as ever.

As to ultra-violet rays, X-rays, etc., keep away from them. Why not get your ray treatment in the natural manner, by an all-over sun bath before the sun gets too high in the morning, or later in the afternoon? Sunlight is beneficial to pyorrhea in all cases, and the use of artificial rays is doubtful, to say the least.

Massage your gums daily with your index finger, having first taken a sufficient amount of lemon juice into the mouth.

RABIES

Q. What is the best thing to do for a mad dog bite?

A. First, tie a bandage between the bite and the heart. Draw it tight enough so that the blood will not go past. Then cauterize with nitrate of silver or a hot iron. Afterward, put the injured member into a mud bath, leaving it there as long as the mud continues to draw. Or you may put on a mud poultice instead.

REFRIGERATION

Q. Does refrigeration impair food value?

A. I do not approve of heavy refrigeration any more than I do of cooking. It is unnatural and destroys food value in greater or lesser degree, depending upon the lowness of the temperature. Grapes, or other fruit, put in refrigeration over night, never taste the same again, but have lost their exotic flavor—in other words, their vito, or life. Certain fruits and vegetables, however, are much more susceptible to low temperature than others. The muscat grape, for instance, is much more delicate in that respect than the Tokay. If you wish really to enjoy your meals and derive the maximum benefit from them, be sure when you purchase your food that you get it sunripened and directly from the fields and orchards.

Live fooders in California need no refrigerators. If you have herbs or roots left over from the preceding day, sprinkle them and set their roots or root-ends in shallow enamel pans. Even a section of watermelon will keep in good condition overnight.

RHEUMATISM AND NEURITIS

Q. Can you tell us why one should be troubled by rheumatism even while living on raw foods?

A. A beginner on raw food will have experiences that are somewhat trying. For instance, the uric acid which has gathered in a crystallized form at the joints, will once more become soluble and be taken up by the blood for transmission to the organs of elimination. Basically, uric acid is the cause of all rheumatism and neuritis. Flesh food is the chief source of this poison. The organs can, under ordinary conditions and without strain, eliminate only three grains of uric acid per day, whereas a pound of meat or fish (and that includes chicken) contains fourteen grains. Liver contains nineteen grains, and sweetbreads seventy per pound. Beef tea is so saturated with uric acid that it can aptly be described as artificial urine. The same is true of chicken broth and other meat extracts.

The body is unable to throw out, as is obvious, the excess of poisonous material in the form of uric acid. Circulating about in the blood stream, it finally comes to rest at the joints and bones in the form of urates, which are solids. You then begin to wonder why your joints are no longer as supple as they were when you were a child, why you cannot run and leap any longer with agility, why even being in a crouching position for a minute or two, seems unbearable. These urates or salts, once deposited, are dormant, in the sense that they no longer move about from one part of the body to another. Under a cooked food régime, however, the system, although not suffering any acute inconvenience by their presence, gradually becomes so heavily loaded with these that a chronic form of suffering, known as rheumatism, or neuritis, gradually appears.

What happens when a sufferer from rheumatism changes to the live food system of living? The urates begin to be dissolved by the action of the alkaline ele· ments, as well as the vito, in the natural food. They are then thrown out again into the bloodstream for elimination, as previously stated. The patient will then suffer, in many cases intensely, will suppose that the food he is eating is the cause of the pains, when in truth it is the dislodging and elimination of the long-stored-up poisons. There can be no cure of a permanent nature unless these are eliminated from the system. While they are on the way out you will suffer acute discomfort, but when the process is completed you will be rid of these pains for all time. Your joints may even become as supple as those of a youth, in time. To hasten the cleaning up, take a blood-heat Epsom salt bath once a day, just before bedtime. Get sunshine on your body (on all of it, not merely a portion); increase the length of your sunbaths as you feel your strength increase.

If, during the periods of crisis, you suffer intense pain, draw blood to the afflicted region by hot applications, followed by a cold sponge. Then exercise, to get the muscles to absorb it.

Q. It is claimed that tomatoes and grapes should not be eaten by those who are afflicted with rheumatism. Is that true?

A. Quite the reverse. Tomatoes and grapes never can create a rheumatic condition. In the first place, they contain no uric acid whatever, and in the second place they are active alkalinizing agents and are therefore natural enemies of all types of destructive acids. In fact, the best foods, in cases of rheumatism and neuritis, are tomatoes, oranges, lemons, and grapefruit. These all contain a certain amount of fruit acid, which, unlike uric acid, is alkalinizing in its effect and beneficial to the human body, and are especially valuable when rheumatic deposits must be loosened up. But always remember that the foods you like best are the ones that are best for you, in disease as well as in health.

RINGWORM

Q. How can you cure ringworm?

A. Ringworm is the result of the expulsion of waste matter from within the body onto the surface of the skin. There it is attacked by various microbes and bacteria that feed on filth. Through their activity, the skin will of course become inflamed and sore within a short time. Basically, ringworm is not different from other forms of skin infection, except that it assumes a characteristic form, round or oval, about the size of a dollar. These eruptions may appear practically anywhere on the body. They are beneficial, and therefore should not be treated by suppressive measures, such as putting on salve and other drug preparations.

When you first begin to eat live food, your ring-worms will not vanish. On the contrary, they very likely will increase in number. Why? Because your system will start to throw off large quantities of stored-up poisons. For some of this, the skin will offer an easy outlet. In a comparatively short time, however, you will find the eruptions all disappearing, sometimes overnight. To reduce the excess inflammation and consequent discomfort, put some lemon juice in a little water, and apply several times a day.

The best foods for skin diseases are fruits. You may have them morning, noon and night, if you wish. Fruits are eliminators by nature.

RUPTURE (HERNIA)

Q. Is hernia curable without operation? If so, tell me how.

A. If you have a hernia on either the left or right side, you must first live from three to six months on natural foods in order to get your blood into good condition, for, if your blood is not right when repairs are made, they will not last. But if you wait until your blood is clean, the repairs will be of good tissue and permanent. At first, then, content yourself by eating raw foods. Toward the end of the period named, get a truss made to fit you. Good fit is essential. Why? Because the button must be in exactly the right place so that when healing commences the cords under it may contract. But we must first inflame these cords by the pressure of the button, irritating as it may be at the time, to get them in contact with each other. Healing tissue will then tie them together by a natural binder, which is elastic and yet efficient. In this manner, the opening is recemented with Nature's own cement. After this process is fairly well completed, you may leave off the truss entirely and forget about it. To test the completeness of the healing, take off the truss, put your hand lightly over the hernia, and cough. If you do not feel anything stirring under your hand, then you will have accomplished your cure. I, myself, have had double hernia and a cardiac rupture besides, and have cured them in the way described.

Q. Why did I rupture myself lifting a heavy weight when two others, not as strong as I, doing the same work, did not?

A. Ruptures are caused by sudden strain in cases where the abdominal muscles are weak or undeveloped. If, by exercise, you had gotten them as strong as those of your partners, likely you would not have suffered a rupture. It should be remarked that you should always try to lift a heavy weight slowly and without jerks or strain.

SALT AND OTHER CONDIMENTS

Q. Would it not be all right to put a little salt on one's food if it seemed to taste "flat" otherwise?

A. Table salt, and all other salts except those found in their organic stages in fruits and vegetables, are inorganic substances which cannot be assimilated by the body and must be discarded by the bloodstream at

the earliest opportunity. Usually the salt is deposited
in the joints, particularly the knees, elbows, ankles,
wrists, and the like, resulting later in arthritis and
rheumatism. It makes no difference whether you have
gotten your salt in the form of the table variety, or as
saleratus (bichloride of soda) in hot biscuits, or
Epsom salts prescribed for internal use in cases of constipation; all are productive of the same injurious results. What is the first symptom of salt deposits in the
joints? Do they crack when you do a knee bend? If
so, your joints are commencing to become dry due to
the salt deposits having absorbed all the synovial fluid
which acts as a lubricant in those regions. Salt has a
tremendous attraction for water and all other liquids.
No wonder doctors prescribe innumerable glasses of
water daily so that their patients may to some extent
satisfy the incessant craving for liquid caused by the
salt they are eating. Remember that salt may dissolve
in water and in the saliva of the mouth, but it will
recrystallize within a very short time and under no
circumstances will it be absorbed into the bodily structure. It will collect wherever there is room for it to be
deposited, but it will no more be absorbed than sand
is absorbed by the gears into which you may have
thrown it. Salt, in its effect, is like that of sand in
gears; it irritates and slowly but surely destroys. Our
bodies are wonderful machines, self-oiling, provided
we furnish the food out of which the oil may be
manufactured and stop abusing them.

You ask, "Do we need salt? Is not salt present in
the healthy bloodstream?" True, but you must get your

salt from the vegetable or fruit, which in turns gets it from the earth. Your bloodstream will not require checking provided you eat natural, uncooked foods. Nature will take from these exactly the right amount of salt which is needed, and no more. In the first place, it is organic, and therefore usable in the building up of the body; in the second place, as mentioned, there will never be an excess of salts no matter how much live food you may eat. Your tastebuds, in their commonly depraved shape, cannot be trusted as to the need for salt of the inorganic type. You say that foods without salt taste "flat." Foods directly from the hands of Nature are never tasteless, but are delicious as only our common Mother knows how to make them. Your tastebuds must be re-educated. They have grown accustomed to the vicious stimulation by the inorganic salt. It may take you some weeks, even months, to get your system adjusted to the new way of living as regards salt, but usually within a very short time your tastebuds will begin to respond to the innumerable subtleties and shadings of flavor even as between bunches of grapes picked from the same vine, between the apples on a single tree, as well as between the several varieties of fruits and vegetables. Nature has made each of us to be a connoisseur of natural flavors, not to be goaded and stabbed into reactions by unnatural condiments.

It is well to remember that more than fifty thousand years are required for molecular change in mineral, crystal salts, but that in organic salt, as in spinach, the change comes once in twenty-four hours. Body cells, having a high rate of molecular change, cannot utilize materials having as low a rate as inorganic salt. This is the reason why inorganic substances cannot be assimilated.

Q. Is it harmful to eat the potato chips found in five or ten cent wax bags? I know of some warranted to be made of sliced raw potatoes.

A. The quality of the food may be determined by the amount of salt required to hide the true flavor or to give it any flavor at all. These chips are crisp only because they have been subjected to a high temperature in frying or other process, thus removing whatever natural taste may reside in the raw potato (and it is a very palatable one) and of course all food value as well. You might as well eat crisp wood shavings. The amount of salt necessary to give the material taste is enormous, but of course the manufacturers and sellers of soft and other drinks will profit correspondingly. Thus you will constantly see these articles together on the same stand. All that has been said applies to salted nuts as well.

Q. Since you say we should not eat inorganic salts, what natural foods are richest in the organic form of sodium chloride?

A. Spinach is rich in this natural element; also beet tops. However, if these do not appeal to your taste, do not eat them—you will find in other foods smaller but appreciable amounts of it.

Q. Taking for granted that salt is no food, why give it to animals?

A. It is well know that cattlemen feed salt to their cattle—that is just why many deaths have been occurring among these animals by hoof and mouth disease. None of the ranchers which had not fed their cattle salt, reported the disease. Moreover, those who had fed salt and stopped doing it, and gave the cattle new pastures, found their animals getting well immediately.

Why do cattle like salt? Domesticated milk cows are constantly given salt for the purpose of getting them thirsty. They will then crave a great deal of water, will distend their stomachs so that they will be able to hold a great deal of grass, and supposedly give a great deal of milk. A dairy cow with its enormously expanded paunch, is an unnatural animal, and can easily acquire, like humans, an unnatural appetite. We must observe these animals under natural conditions before we venture to say cattle naturally like or must have salt.

Why is it that elk and deer will go to the salt lick once or twice a year? The elk or deer must guard itself against beasts of prey, such as bears, wolves, mountain lions. Therefore, the instinct of the elk leads him to avoid coughing. Once or twice a year the elk renews the inner membrane of its throat. Because it eats grass and other natural foods, the membranes are very strong, and when these are loosened, they tickle the throat, causing a cough. Now, the salt will hasten the breaking up of this membrane so that all of the loosening substance will come out at once. However, the salt that the elk gets is rock salt, not our common salt which is charged with chloroform gas. This rock salt is hardly salty at all, compared with our salt, and besides, they can get but very little, it being very hard.

Q. Is cinnamon healthful? Should one use it at all?

A. Use cinnamon for influenza. Use it, then, on fruit, if you like. It is not necessary to season live foods. As regards seasoning value, the addition of flavor to food, the same applies to other spices and aromatic herbs, such as nutmeg, ginger, cloves, allspice, mustard, pepper, paprika, sage, and thyme. When your tastebuds have become normalized, you will not need to add any seasoning to your food. The combinations you make will become simpler and simpler as time goes on and your tastebuds develop their original vigor. In the end, you will enjoy a meal of a single type of food, or a simple combination of two, more than any complex mixtures for which your mouth now waters. A transition period, to be sure, is often found necessary, but constant effort should be made to work toward the true, natural diet. If you feel like eating some cinnamon powder, eat some, but eat it alone. Since it is a bark and a natural product, it will then be a natural food. If your tastebuds crave the pepper flavor, eat some of the pepper from the can as it comes to you, or get one of the vegetable peppers found in the markets. Your craving will soon be gratified, and may not recur.

Q. Is it safe to use canned spices?

A. Fresh vegetable spices, such as peppers, garlic, onions, are in every case to be preferred. Do not buy

ground spices: you do not know what you are getting.
Grind your own.

Q. Is brown sugar suitable to use as a sweetener?
How about molasses and maple syrup?

A. Brown sugar is not a natural product, as it has
been heated in the process of extraction, and has later
been refined somewhat. Brown sugar is more natural
than white sugar, but it is not a desirable sweetener for
human food. The same is true of molasses. Maple
syrup is boiled to death and is not to be recommended
as an article of diet. And while we're at it, we may add
corn syrup to this category.

Q. Do you recommend kelp in place of table salt?
It is said to contain many valuable elements necessary
to the human body.

A. There is one thing to be said for kelp. Although
it is saturated with inorganic sea salt, an unassimilable
compound of elements, it does contain much organic
iodine, a rare and precious element of our diet. It is
known that the constant absence of iodine from the
food we eat causes goitre and allied diseases. Goitre is
particularly prevalent in regions far from the sea, as
for instance our own Upper Mississippi Valley. Near
the sea coast, however, as here on the Pacific slope,
there appears to be much free iodine in the soil, particularly in areas immediately contiguous to the ocean.
Now, plants that grow in the soil of the Upper Mississippi Valley have no iodine in them because there is
none in the soil, whereas those fruits and vegetables
which are grown near the sea have distinct traces of it,

sufficient for the body's needs. Then, why not forget about the smelly, salt-saturated kelp, a thing which no normal tastebud yet ever craved, and eat instead vegetables grown in soil rich in iodine? It may be possible to supply iodine to the soil where it is lacking at present, through the addition of ground kelp as fertilizer. When this is done, as experiments seem to indicate, there is a true trace of iodine in the resulting crops.

So much for the real value of kelp, or, rather, its constituent, iodine. As to a substitute for table salt, the sea salt always found in it is not a whit better than the refined variety, considered as human food. Keep away from it.

SAUERKRAUT

Q. Is uncooked sauerkraut a good food?

A. Sauerkraut is commonly prepared by the use of salt, and is therefore dead as far as life-giving qualities are concerned. Salt always destroys life. Sauerkraut is liked by many because it tickles their tastebuds, and not because their system naturally craves it. When tastebuds are covered with phlegm, they will seem to call for all sorts of perverted foods. It is necessary to remove the phlegm in order to make these organs trustworthy. Meanwhile, we must use our reasoning power in determining which foods are best for us.

Sauerkraut is fermented cabbage, in the preparation of which salt is used. Furthermore, sauerkraut is in an early state of decay. We may think that salt is preserving it from bacterial action, but fermentation itself is bacterial activity. Sauerkraut is not natural cabbage in any sense of the word, but a putrefying substance held in suspension for a time by the action of salt.

It makes no difference whether you cook sauerkraut or whether you eat it as it comes from the market—the results are the same. It will cause hardening of the arteries, which in the end means apoplexy. Sauerkraut juice is just as bad as the kraut itself since it is simply a by-product of fermentation. Even supposing salt has not been added, an unnatural product like this will never lead to health—just the reverse. If you feel you would like cabbage soured a bit, shred, and add rhubarb juice. Let it stand for several hours before eating. Such natural cabbage is good for constipation. The fermented product will cause more harm than good in the long run.

SEASICKNESS

Q. What is the cause and cure of seasickness? Some get seasick very easily whereas others never do.

A. Being on the ocean or any other large body of water, especially during a storm, is unnatural. You might enjoy a good sail on smooth waters, but certainly your powers of observation should have been called upon in time to prevent your being caught out in heavy weather. Sea gulls and other sea fowl are always inshore in case of storm. A storm at sea is an emergency, and as such it will test the endurance of the human body. Being tossed about on a ship taxes the powers of resistance. If any organs are by nature weak, they will suffer. With many of us, the stomach is the first to give way. It finds it impossible to digest food when the vital forces of the body are being employed in combating the effects of the unusual environment. The most obvious cure for seasickness is to stop eating. Live fooders will not be as apt to suffer from seasickness as cooked fooders. If you are much in the open air, that will help to stabilize your stomach at the time. It is as much a matter of general physical vitality as anything else. Live fooders, in this regard, have a tremendous advantage over others since they will have stored up a great fund of vitality, and furthermore, the food they eat will be very easy to digest. An acid state of the body is the predisposing cause of seasickness as well as other illness. Steamship companies, when they furnish their passengers with slices of lemon, show a vague intuition of the true cause and cure of the trouble. With sensitive people, fear sometimes causes the stomach to become unbalanced—fear, particularly of deep water and unstable footing, being out of sight of land, etc. These persons are proverbially poor sailors.

SEX

Q. Is it true that if one lives on a raw food diet, one eventually loses sexual desires?

A. No, this is not true. While you are being reconstructed, that is the way you will feel at the start, but do not be alarmed. After some months, or a year, your sexual organism will be stronger than ever, but not as excitable. Cooked fooders, and especially meat eaters, suffer from over-stimulation of the sex glands. Nature seems to feel death on the way, and is in a hurry to reproduce while there is yet time. The excess acids in the system irritate the glands, make them seem very strong, when, as a matter of fact, they are very weak, are operating at high tension. This, prolonged over a period of time, will cause them to degenerate and stop functioning entirely, as often happens with persons over forty who for many years have been abusing their powers.

Sex is by nature for reproduction only, and is therefore not intended to be used constantly and promiscuously. These glands are also created for the purpose of furnishing hormones to the blood, which, when present in abundance, will enable us to think and act intelligently, to feel vital in our everyday activities, and to develop ourselves in the many varied fields as Nature intended we should do. When we constantly waste our sex fluid, we shall have little vigor left for our daily activities.

With the huge amount of specialized activity in our so-called civilized life, there seems to be little time left for purposes of well-rounded development. But it is only by thus developing the whole being, and not simply the body, or the mind, alone, that we can avoid unnatural desires, such as the craving for constant sex contacts and adventures. These are inevitably associated with a degenerating society, luxurious and effeminate, and never with a virile and truly masculine one.

Q. Is menstruation a normal function in women? I understand it is considered by some an unnatural result of our unnatural life.

A. It is an entirely normal activity of the female

organism, but the unpleasant symptoms now considered part and parcel of it will, when the woman lives naturally, disappear. This may take some time, since the entire body must be rebuilt time after time until it has reached a sufficiently high degree of perfection. The symptoms spoken of are merely one form of elimination, the casting out of the body accumulated waste poisons. So long as there are any of these resident in the body, you will to some degree suffer the consequences.

Q. How can a man regain his lost potency?

A. First, let him stop wastage of the vital forces, by the less as well as the more obvious channels. Not only should he be sexually continent, but loss of energy by excess expenditure of nervous force in mental overwork; hyperstimulation, as in city life, and the like, should be guarded against. Not only should he guard well what he already possesses; he should also labor earnestly to build up a reserve fund of the fluid of life. This can be done through faithful following of the natural life routine. Be thrifty and save, in a moral and physical, as well as a financial way. If you draw constantly upon the bank of health and strength, without making deposits, your checks will some day be returned, marked "no funds."

SINUS TROUBLE

Q. What causes sinus trouble, and how should one go about curing it?

A. Accumulations of waste matter in that region are the primary cause. All kinds of infection come only because of waste matter present. No bacteria will ever remain active in your body unless there is something for them to eat and to breathe in. All are scavengers, Nature's broom. When you live on natural foods, the waste matter is removed and the trouble is automatically dispelled.

Use hot applications, alternating with cold, over the sinus area, and you will be much relieved immediately. Spray the nose with finely strained lemon juice several times daily if there is too much soreness. The lemon juice destroys pus. Do not use drug store preparations or antiseptics. They are harmful in every instance and are only temporary palliatives at best. Often the membranes are weakened by their use and become less resistant to germ infection than they were before. Operations are of no value, of course.

SKIN—CARE OF THE

Q. May fruit or vegetable juice, instead of soap, be used for washing the human body? Would it be as cleansing?

A. The morning cold shower or cold water rubdown may be taken without the use of soap, and lemon juice or orange juice applied over the body with the hands, either before or after washing. The juice will smooth and whiten the skin, is a good dirt chaser, disinfectant, and also will act as a mild astringent. Soaps often contain caustics; even those made of vegetable oils have a tendency to dry the skin, but orange or lemon juice have no harmful effects. Housekeepers will find good use for their lemon rinds in cleaning and whitening the hands when they are soiled. Just a few drops of the juice are necessary. After shampooing the hair, lemon juice, mixed with the last rinsing water, will soften both the water and the hair. You may use the juices with as good effect after washing as before. After the shower or bath, rub your body down with the juice of half an orange or lemon while the skin is still moist. Massage gently until perfectly dry—otherwise the skin will have a tendency to be somewhat sticky, especially with oranges. This massage will work the dirt out of the pores and also dislodge outworn skin. With the slightly astringent effect, you will feel clean and be clean after it is over. Only a few minutes are required.

Q. Do you recommend the use of cold cream or vaseline?

A. Vaseline is a coal tar product, and as such it should certainly not be used internally. It may, however, be applied externally, in case of emergency, to prevent chapping of the skin, sunburn, and the like; yet, being processed, it is an unnatural agent. Why not use a fruit or vegetable preparation such as is sold at health food stores, or a mixture of olive oil and lemon juice, or even the fruit or vegetable juices alone?

Q. Is it possible to get rid of freckles?

A. Excessive freckles mean that you have a fair skin which does not tan easily. Freckles are usually an indication that there is plenty of iron in your blood, which is a good sign. Nature doubtless makes freckles appear for some definite reason, possibly to protect the skin. However, if you wish to remove the freckles, you may bathe them with clabbered milk, applied for a couple of hours. Do this several times, and you will be rid of them—not permanently, however.

Q. What foods are good for the complexion?

A. All natural foods, particularly dried olives, beets, carrots, and apples, as these contain much natural pigment.

Q. Do you endorse commercial shaving creams? Also, is the styptic pencil, used to stop the bleeding of shaving cuts, injurious?

A. Under our present economic system, it is practically impossible for the average person to know of, or detect, the presence of injurious chemicals in commercial creams. All inorganic chemicals applied to the skin are harmful. For instance, the humus found in the soil, wiped on the skin in the form of mud, is rather beneficial than otherwise. It is not a part of the inorganic rock, which merely serves as binder, but is decayed organic vegetable matter, which has astringent and often alkaline effects, depending upon its cleanness and other factors. Therefore, use only such shaving creams as are compounded one hundred per cent of fruit and vegetable elements. Vegetable soap can be lathered with a brush and applied, with splendid results. The lather may seem a little light, but you will notice that the beard softens beautifully under additional application. Sayman's is a good and popular brand.

Styptic pencils are composed of highly poisonous

caustics, inorganic in nature as a rule. Use, instead, a cold application sustained long enough to cause the blood to withdraw from that area and enable a clot to form and the cut edges to unite. If you think there is any danger of infection, use orange or lemon juice as antiseptics.

Q. How can I best get rid of the wrinkles on my face?

A. These so-called "crow's-feet" of time are really a confession to all who can read, of health and strength ill spent, of a life lived out of accord with Nature. What, then, is the remedy? The Bible says there is no sin that shall not be forgiven provided you repent and sin no more. That holds good in the physical as well as the moral world. Change your habits of living, and you will see the wrinkles fade out with the advent of your new body.

On the other hand, exposure wrinkles, caused by undue impact of wind and weather upon sensitive skin, are sometimes not entirely avoidable. Anoint your face with some good vegetable or fruit oil before going out of doors, also upon coming back at night. Orange juice, too, is good.

SKIN DISEASES

Q. What is acne?

A. Acne is a skin disease which many people get for the first time when they come to this semi-tropical country and eat plenty of oranges and other citrus fruits. It is a disease of the sebaceous glands of the skin, which secrete a fatty substance which serves as a lubricant for the exterior surface. Since fresh fruit is very plentiful and cheap here in California, newcomers often eat it in much larger quantity than that to which they have been accustomed in less favored climates. The poisons which have accumulated in their bodies through the years suddenly get stirred up and are exuded through the skin in the form of pimples, rash, and like skin afflictions, as well as through the lungs, colon, and kidneys. One form of such elimination is called "acne." It is annoying, but necessary, considering the condition your body is in. You can reduce the irritation by swabbing the areas affected with a solution of lemonized water, perhaps half and half in strength. Do not be alarmed when the lemon burns you at the beginning; this is a beneficial activity of the alkaline element in the juice. It will pass and take with it the itching sensation of the skin. After a short while, you may have to repeat the operation. Thus you may disinfect and cleanse the skin and destroy the pus formations around the glands.

Do not think that it is the oranges, lemons, or grapefruit you have eaten that are the primary cause of your trouble. They are merely the house servants of Nature, which, through them, is cleansing the poisons from your body. Naturally, during the time that they are at work, you will suffer inconvenience and discomfort, but the way you will feel after it is all over will more than compensate you. Do not stop eating these fruits when the acne appears: rather, continue and encourage Nature in her beneficent activities. As time goes on, you will be able to enjoy increasing resistance to all aerial bacteria, such as those which are feeding on the waste exuded from the skin and contribute to that characteristic inflammatory appearance and itching feeling. These bacteria are scavengers like worms that feed on barnyard manure. If you use lemon juice, you will accomplish the same beneficent end that they do, and with much less irritation to yourself.

Q. What causes eczema, and how can you cure it?

A. Eczema tells of a large amount of waste matter in the body. It is a catarrhal refuse breaking out through the skin. Aerial germs come in large numbers and feed upon this refuse, thus, as you see, eliminating it, but slowly, and without much pleasure to the patient. The most fundamental cure is to clean the inside rather than the outside of your body, although both are necessary. First of all you should adopt a natural diet. In the second place, you should bathe frequently, exercise, and expose yourself for a short time daily to the sunshine. Do not overdo the sunbathing, however. Salves are of no value; on the contrary, most of them contain injurious drugs which suppress the poisons, preventing them from coming out. What you want is to have them eliminated as easily and rapidly as possible. Lemon or orange juice applications to the affected parts are of value in relieving the irritation by neutralizing the exuding acids. Put on as often as necessary.

Q. What is pellagra?

A. Pellagra is an eruption very commonly found in southern climates, as for instance in Italy and in our own southern states. It is found where much salt pork and like valueless foods are eaten. Being a deficiency disease, it is easily remedied by supplying the proper elements and vito-energy, as found in fresh fruits and vegetables. Pellagra is considered incurable by the bulk of the medical profession, but there is no incurable disease. All that is required is to give Nature a chance to clean out and rebuild the body according to her own specifications. Insect bites, said by some to cause pellagra, are nothing more than an easy way out, a specious explanation for the use of doctors who really know nothing about the true cause of disease. As in the case of the mosquito's relation to malaria, insect bites as a true cause of pellagra are a joke. If the body were healthy, there would be no unfavorable reaction, bite or no bite. A mucous-filled body, on the other hand, will begin severe eliminations on slight provocation. That is only Nature's way of cleaning and scouring.

Q. What causes a widespread rash over arm and body? I got it after eating live food for four weeks.

A. A rash always means waste matter circulating in the body bloodstream, that it is being poured out through the skin and there devoured by minute, irritative organisms. The live food you have been eating has been stirring up material that should have been removed long ago. It is going out through your kidneys, bowels, and lungs, as well as through your skin. Keep on eating whatever of live food appeals most to your taste. As Hippocrates said, "Your food shall be your remedy." Observe the rules of cleanliness within as well as outside your body, conserve your energy, get plenty of fresh air and sunshine, particularly on the affected parts. However, if the eruption is too troublesome or too long drawn out, you can always reduce it by eating less of the eliminative fruits and more of the building vegetables, especially roots.

Q. Please tell me about inflammation of the skin, and the cure.

A. If you fall or slide on a rough floor or other hard surface, where the skin makes contact you will invariably find some form of inflammation within a short time after. The blood rushes to the area, causing temporary congestion. Apply lemon juice diluted in warm or cold water. This will allay the inflammation, as lemon is one of the most powerful disinfectants we have, and an absolutely natural one, created by action of the sun, air, and water upon earth elements.

Q. What is the value of cocoa butter for itching skin or scalp?

A. Although cocoa butter is better used outside than inside the body, its value is slight. Wherever an oily lotion is of benefit, I would recommend not cocoa butter, which is processed, but pure olive or almond oil. For itch, instead, use some fruit juice, diluted in water if you wish.

Q. My skin is becoming chapped and sore. What can I do for this?

A. There is too much acid still in your body, seeking elimination through the skin. If it is your hands that are affected, wash them with a good vegetable soap; then rub in some olive oil or orange juice. Do this also whenever you have exposed your hands or face to the unfavorable conditions which caused them to chap. Some skin is by nature delicate and easily broken. It requires protection from extremes of humidity and temperature. Usually such protection is furnished by the natural oils, but if for any reason they are absent, you must supply them yourself. After a time your skin may function normally, or you may find it possible to avoid the unfavorable environment. Natural living, of course, is a prerequisite.

Q. I have a brown patch about an inch in diameter on my right arm. What is the cause and cure of this? It is not a liver spot. I bruised myself there several months ago.

A. You very likely have poor circulation, as well as poor blood, or the discoloration would have disappeared long ago. Nature is in the habit of cleaning up all repair work as rapidly as she can. The average individual of today has difficulty in finding enough energy for his daily work, let alone elimination of unusual conditions or disease. Your blood is your own best healer, but first it must be made potent by eating the proper foods—live, not soggy, dead foods. In my practice, I have never noticed the condition you suffer from on any live fooder.

As for treatment, apply hot water to the spot until there is a plentiful supply of blood present in the region of the injury. With your hand, stroke the blood away from the spot and upwards, following the veinous circulation. Do this until the blood has all been forced away—twice a day at least.

Q. I have brown spots all over my body. Are they called liver spots?

A. Evidently some form of unassimilated pigmentation is in your blood and being thrown off through the skin. It makes little difference what you call the spots —they are simply caused by the elimination of useless pigment. You have been eating, perhaps, a great deal of cooked vegetables, like carrots, beets, spinach, red cabbage, as well as strawberries, blackberries, and like highly colored fruits. All these things when eaten un· cooked will never trouble you in any way as the pigmentation is easily assimilated or passed off if all is not needed. But when cooked, there is a different tale to tell. We vainly expect our blood to use such dead coloring matter in the construction of tissue.

Q. What could be done for a yellow skin? I live quite naturally.

A. Yellowish skin (often called jaundice) is due to discharge of excess bile from the gall bladder. Your liver is working overtime and producing more bile than you can use. This feverish activity, in turn, may be due to a habit formed while eating denatured foods. For instance, a small piece of fried beeksteak would not call on the bile to any extent, but if you immediately afterwards take helpings of boiled or mashed potatoes, bile will be demanded by the body in overdoses. Thus the liver gets overworked habitually. This habit has been formed in past time and the liver is still functioning that way in spite of your eating more normal food, and it may continue to do so for some time. The excess of bile, of course, gets into the blood and thence into the skin, making it yellow.

Exercise your liver by using stretching and other movements that are designed for that purpose. Use plenty of olive oil or the sun-dried olives themselves; also avocados. They will help lubricate the gall duct and stabilize the demand for bile. Put hot applications over the liver when you feel distressed or uncomfortable. Give yourself a hot and cold shower daily. That will help the skin to eliminate. Eat plenty of grapes, oranges, and leafy vegetables, according to taste. Take Epsom salt baths once or twice a week.

Q. What can be done for blackheads? My skin is much too oily also, particularly around the nose.

A. Steam your face thoroughly with a hot bath towel, and when there is plenty of blood below the skin surface, rub on some lemon juice. Do this for three or four days. Then, with the aid of a vegetable soap, scrub your face thoroughly, using a rough cloth, especially around the nose. The blackheads will come out readily under such treatment. Then give another steaming, with the lemon rub following. Your mirror will tell you of your success.

Excess oil on the skin is caused by overworked oil glands. When your body is in better condition these glands will do their work in a more normal manner. Lemon, and in fact all fruit juices, tend to remove anv present over supply.

Q. What would you do for a case of hives?

A. Hives, too, are caused by elimination of waste matter from the body by means of the skin. They are a blessing in disguise, although they cause plenty of discomfort at the time. If the patient is a child, see that it gets plenty of sleep, fresh air, and sunshine, removing all excess clothing. To reduce the inflammation, use lemon juice in water, applied frequently. If an adult, be careful not to over-exert yourself, since Nature has, at such a time, plenty of work to do.

Q. I have outcroppings of psoriasis periodically. I am a 100 per cent live fooder. What can be done for this skin affliction?

A. You apparently still have plenty of waste matter in your system. You should be glad it is coming out. Do not, however, overeat of eliminative food. To reduce the inflammation of the affected areas, use cold water packs numerous times daily; also lemon juice as a disinfectant.

SLEEP

Q. I sleep about five hours every night. Is that enough?

A. That depends upon your age; the older you are, the less sleep you require. Children up to fifteen should sleep nine or ten hours each night. Those from fifteen to thirty should sleep at least eight hours every night, and those over thirty should adjust their sleeping hours to their individual needs. In general, we may say that a feeling of weariness indicates the need for sleep. A live fooder should be alert and vigorous throughout his waking hours. If he is not, it is a sign that something is wrong, and as likely as not this condition will be benefited by more sleep than he is in the habit of getting. The night hours are intended by Nature for recuperation and rest — not for stimulating amusements. If then, you are over thirty, five hours may be sufficient, if your feelings do not indicate otherwise.

Q. What is the cause of desire for sleep at inconvenient times, as, for instance, when we want to stay awake to see a show or hear a lecture?

A. After you have been living on live food for some time, you will begin to feel this craving for rest, for that is what it is—time out to repair and reconstruct. Everyone should get all the sleep he craves. The bodies of those of us who have lived on cooked foods for many years, are desperately in need of, first, elimination, next, reconstruction. During the period of elimination, the veins are full of waste matter moving toward the organs of expulsion, as lungs, kidneys, the bowels, and skin. This process requires much energy. Those of us who work all day long need, particularly in eliminative periods, as much sleep as we can get. It would be wise, if you feel like it, to spend the entire Sunday holiday in bed. Nature will appreciate the lift, and you will be well all the sooner for it. Natural foods do not merely aid in elimination, but of course also in reconstruction. They are full of vito (life) and organic mineral matter. When your body has been cleansed sufficiently, it will be gradually rebuilt into the form and energy you possessed in youth.

Patience is required, and sleeping, too, has its rewards, though you may seem inactive and even lazy for the nonce. Sleepiness, then, is just an indication that your working day's activities are at an end. It is as much a mandate of Nature, to be disobeyed at your peril, as the call for food.

Q. Is sleep necessary to health? What do you think of the value of short naps in the middle of the day or at other times during daylight hours?

A. When you feel drowsy, the best thing to do is to lie down on a cot or on the grass for five or ten minutes. Just a few minutes will make a great deal of difference in the way you feel. Even a one or two minute cat-nap is a good thing whenever you feel like taking one. Some gymnasts often, when tired in between periods of their daily training, drop off to sleep for a few minutes. They do this because they feel themselves much benefited. Muscle and nerve tension are both relieved. Often a nap makes one feel as fresh as in the early morning hours. The blood gets a chance to dispose of its excess burden of waste material, and more energy is available for other necessary activity. Yes, sleep is necessary, and in the quantities for which your body indicates desire.

Q. Please tell me what causes insomnia and what the best remedy is.

A. Insomia is not a matter forr jesting, but indicates a very serious state of bodily affairs. Nerves, and even mind, may be affected by its long continuance. Many victims of chronic insomnia commit suicide;

others take to drugs for relief, or alcoholic beverages, and find therein a deadly trap instead of that which is promised. I myself some years ago handled the case of a doctor who had become a dope fiend through the torture of insomnia. I had to follow him like a detective during the first few weeks, to be sure that he carried out my directions. But after a comparatively short period he was completely cured, of both insomnia and the craving for drugs. What performed this seeming miracle? Live food, coupled with natural living. After he became well, there were no more cocktails on his table, but plenty of raw salads and vegetable juices.

Insomnia is a disease where the nerves are in such a state of tension that they will not allow you to sleep at night, or, for that matter, to function normally in the daytime. Sometimes patients are afraid to go to sleep for fear they will not wake up in the morning. This indicates a definitely diseased nervous organism. As to cause, some doctors ascribe all this to poor blood circulation, but it is really due to constant violation of Nature's laws, both in the matter of food and in the rest of our daily routine of living. Food which is cooked is unable to furnish the nerves with assimilable material for repair or rebuilding.

As a temporary aid toward restoring normal sleep, try the water cure. It consists of immersion of your entire body into a lukewarm bath, not hot and not cold—just a sleep-conveying tepidness. Have at the bottom of your tub, to recline on, a woolen blanket. After you have been in the bath for twenty minutes to half an hour, you will commence to get drowsy. When this feeling comes on, get out, wrap a dry blanket tightly about you, and go to bed, blanket and all. The blanket will absorb the moisture from your body, as well as stimulate the skin sufficiently to induce semi-hypnotic influence in the direction of sleep. You will be surprised how easily you will drop off. Be sure not to use a towel after this bath or to put on pajamas— get directly into the blanket and bed. Keep plenty of covers over you.

Q. What foods are best for one suffering from insomnia?

A. Do not drink any sort of liquid just before retiring. In fact, allow three hours to elapse between the last meal-time and bedtime. That will allow all foods to be digested before sleep begins. Your nerves will be settled and good dreams, if any, will be in order.

If possible, have your evening meal a simple one, although as plentiful in quantity as you may desire. Eat onions with the rest of your food in the evening, either green ones or the large bulb variety.

Q. Is it best to sleep with one's head toward the north or east?

A. It makes no difference whether your head is toward the north or south, provided you sleep comfortably and awake refreshed. I have experimented with this considerably and have found absolutely no difference. So with sleeping on any particular side. Although there may be some slight benefit in lying on your right side as far as your heart action is concerned, it is practically negligible. If it agrees with you to sleep on your right side, do so. On the other hand, if you have a preference for your left side, or, for that matter, the back or the stomach, lie that way. You will be able to judge by results and allow them to determine your choice.

Q. Is there any advantage in sleeping on the ground?

A. Yes, you get in direct contact with the earth and its magnetic vibrations, soothing and invigorating to the tired body. You will awake after a night spent on the ground (suitably covered, of course) feeling much more refreshed than you would from a night spent in a bed, even one placed directly on the ground. Camping, for this reason, is a health-giving form of recreation. Leave your patented sleeping apparatus at home, however. Avoid, especially, all rubber fabrics between you and the earth, since these are non-conductive and shut off the direct currents from below.

Some say that we should sleep, in a house or apartment building, preferably on the lower floors, for the most restful sleep, since the earth currents find most of our modern flimsy building material a non-conductor, which would not be true if it were substantial stone, brick, or concrete.

Q. Would you advise us to sleep on a blanket on the floor, rather than in a soft bed?

A. Several moving picture actresses, famed for their beauty and vitality, habitually sleep on hard pallets, even directly on the floor or hard ground. They have found that the secret of a refreshing sleep lies not in the softness of the mattress and springs, but in the ability of the nerves and muscles to completely relax. Oftentimes when we lie in a fluffy bed, we think we are having a peaceful rest, that the body has lost its day time tension, and that all is well. In truth, this is usually not the case at all; the bed yields and the nerves do not, but remain rigid and impressionable. Now, on a hard bed, if you wish to get any sleep at all, you will have to relax, often consciously, and keep relaxed all night long. So much for the primal purpose of most city dwellers' sleep. Furthermore, soft beds as a rule mean poor posture: a forward-bent upper trunk with a flat chest, prominent buttocks and abdomen. In the harder type of bed, you are forced to assume a natural breathing position, which is invaluable, particularly when lying on your back.

In choosing your type of bed, it is wise to remember that there is a golden mean between bare boards and featherbeds. Even animals are inclined to build themselves ground nests of leaves or other soft material. We should use our judgment, making the bed just hard enough, and inflexible enough, for the best results, without indulging a martyr complex too much. Then circulation will not be impeded, which is sometimes the case when the bed is too rigid and straight. A thin pad or blanket will do, between body and resting spot.

Q. Some people say that pillows are bad for posture. Is that true?

A. Yes, throw away your pillows. If you must have something under your head, make it a thin blanket folded up once or twice.

Q. My two daughters, aged ten and fifteen years, share the same bed. Is this harmful to either or both of them?

A. Children, particularly when approaching the adolescent age, should always sleep without the necessity of physical contact with others of any age whatever. It is a fairly well substantiated fact that the weaker of the two individuals will drain off the surplus energy of the stronger. Nature, in this way, tends to equalize the distribution of strength. In some cases, this is legitimate, as when a mother sleeps with her baby enfolded in her arms. Sick or weak persons are known to be benfited by the mere application of hands by one endowed with a nervous energy easily tapped. The hands act, in this case, as conductors. But growing children particularly should never be in physical contact with another during hours of rest.

SNAKE BITES

Q. What is your remedy for rattlesnake bites?

A. Place a bandage between the bite and the heart. If on the leg, tie below or above the knee, and tighten by twisting with a stick. Next, make an incision with a sharp knife, and suck the wound, expectorating the poison. If there is an open sore in the mouth of the person bitten, have someone else do the sucking, if possible. If you have a lemon with you, mash some of the pulp on a bandage, and apply. The prime essential is to keep the poison away from the heart, and these simple devices will accomplish that end quite thoroughly if you lose no time. Or, if you have no lemon, take some water out of your canteen and moisten sufficient earth to make a semi-liquid mud poultice, which you can then apply in place of the fruit pulp. Keep it moist and leave on for several hours, at least. Should there be a pool of water nearby, with a mud bottom, do not be afraid to bury the injured member right in the mud. I have seen pigs bitten by rattlesnakes go into a mud hole, bury their bites, and come out perfectly cured; no ill effects visible. Horses bitten in the legs can also be saved in this manner. In these cases where the wound comes into direct contact with the earth, there is much more effective action—the magnetism of the earth acts in conjunction with the chemical constituents of the soil to draw out the snake poison from the tissues. If you should be bitten by a snake, do not become frightened. Above all, do not start running. Rather, sit down in the shade after you have given yourself emergency treatments, and relax for several hours. The safety-kit or serum type of treatment is never to be advised. To fight poison by adding more poison is worse than senseless. You may permanently injure your heart by so doing.

SPRAINS AND STRAINS

Q. What is good for a sprained ankle?

A. Put your ankle immediately into hot water, just as hot as possible, and keep it that way for at least half an hour. Do not touch the injured part at all, but stroke, with the flat of your hand, just above it, upward toward the knee. Keep on doing this as long as you have your foot in the water. In that manner, you will force the used-up blood away from the injured part, allowing the new arterial blood with its load of healing elements, to come. It will then in turn take away its load of impurities as you keep stroking, and soon you will find that soreness and inflammation have disappeared. This process may take you from a half hour to an hour and a half, but carry on. When you feel that the ankle has become normal again, remove from the hot water and for two or three minutes immerse it into a cold bath. Then wrap a dry bath towel around it and give it a rest until morning, when you will be able to walk as though nothing had happened. If you have a sprain of long standing, treat it in the same manner every day until the swelling is gone. You will not be able to reduce the swelling in one operation, as it will have commenced to set.

Stroking the leg in the manner described hurries the blood on its way to the heart, from where it is pumped into the lungs. These organs throw off the impurities. Then, by oxidation, the blood is restored to normalcy and carries healing material to the sprain. I suggest hot, rather than cold, water because hot water attracts blood whereas cold water keeps it away. Your blood is your best healing agent.

This same treatment applies to a strained shoulder, sprained wrist, hip, or whatever the case may be. You may have to apply the heat by means of hot towels.

STAMMERING

Q. What can one do for stammering?

A. The first thing you must do is to cleanse your

blood, for it is full of poison. Your nerves have gone to pieces, and you will notice that at times your whole body is atremble. Jangling nerves need to be fed. Uncooked food will do it. After your blood gets into good condition through natural living, take some singing exercises. Singing will help cure stammering. There is a logical and very likely true story concerning a boy stammerer who one day excitedly rushed out of the house and tried, without success, to tell something to his father, who was some distance away. He tried many times but could not utter a word. Finally, the father exclaimed, "Sing it." The boy sang, "Father, oh father, our house is on fire!" A stammerer can always sing. Let your patient repeat a melody after you in sing-song fashion for fifteen or twenty minutes. You may vary the tune if you like. Continue this daily until the fault disappears. Although poor health is the basic cause, habit also is a considerable factor. By the aid of rhythm the primitive speech centers can be brought into renewed activity and the stammerer may learn to speak, as it were, all over again. He has gotten into a bad habit. It must be broken and a natural habit must supplant it. He must learn to control himself, since stammering is chronic lack of control over the vocal cords.

STOMACH DISORDERS

Q. Can a person with stomach trouble eat too much honey?

A. Stomach trouble or none, you can eat too much honey as well as too much of anything else. Your stomach is not a storehouse. It is not necessary to eat enough in one day for the rest of your life. Your stomach is intended to handle only enough food to keep you for a few hours or until your next meal. It is merely a digestive organ, not a repository. How can you tell when you have eaten enough? You will feel satisfied and yet not bulky or overly full. Do not feel unduly alarmed, however, because your appetite is large. Your body, starved for many years, is clamoring for the real food you are furnishing it. As your body becomes rebuilt, your appetite will diminish, sometimes very quickly, especially after a crisis or acute cleansing period.

Q. Please give the treatment for prolapsed stomach and colon.

A. Do not eat great quantities, but rather in small doses. You may eat just as much, but spread it out. Eat every three or four hours, or every hour if you must. Hunger is the signal. If you eat until your stomach is full, the contents sometimes will not be properly digested. Your stomach may be weak and require especially considerate treatment. Prolapsis means that your organs have been stretched out of their natural shape. Therefore, when you take small quantities only, they will gradually, as they work over the material, come back to their normal size and position. Your big stomach will change into a normal one, approximately the size of your doubled fist, when full. You will be hungry practically all the time for a while, but don't let that worry you. The habit of overeating needs to be broken and the stomach repaired. All this causes a feeling of discomfort. Allow as long a time to elapse between meals as you can. Any exercises that bring the muscles over the abdomen and stomach into play, will help your rejuvenation. They need not be stereotyped, but should be vigorous and practiced daily without fail.

Q. Is it possible for one with gastritis to start in immediately eating one hundred per cent raw foods? I have found that nuts and grains disagree with me; even certain salads.

A. The cause of gastritis is the eating of fermentable foods. All cooked foods and dairy products, also many uncooked fruits and vegetables (including legumes), are fermentable. There is, however, a vast difference between the ferment of uncooked fruits and vegetables and that of cooked foods and dairy products. Cooked foods produce a heavy, sour ferment, very oppressive and hence dangerous. The fruits and vegetables, however, produce a light, sweet ferment, embarrassing, perhaps, but never dangerous. If you suffer from gastritis, it would be well to eat certain non-fermentable natural foods. These are: greens, as lettuce, cabbage, cauliflower, asparagus, water cress, endive, rhubarb, dandelion, sorrel, parsley, mustard greens, nasturtium leaves. The roots as a class are non-fermentable. Here you have a wide choice: Irish and sweet potatoes, carrots, turnips, beets, parsnips, radishes, rutabagas, ground artichokes, celery root, and the like. You may eat as much of these non-fermentable foods as you desire, singly or in combination, and you will suffer no ill effect. It is better to eat them singly than in complex mixtures, in order to make the work of digestion easier. You should also see that they are fresh, taken, if possible, directly from the garden or ranch. A caution, however, is in order; namely, that you may find gas in your stomach coming not from the food which you have eaten, but from the phlegm which has been loosened there or in the connecting tubes. What shall you do about this? Keep right on eating these foods which stir up the long-settled poisons. You will feel uncomfortable for a while, but do not fear. It will not be for long. The raw Irish potatoes are especially valuable, as well as ground artichokes, in such cases, provided always that you like them.

Some general hints—depend upon your own saliva for digestion. In other words, do not drink anything with your meals, and allow to half an hour before and two hours after for the digestive juices to function without dilution from outside sources. If your stomach is inflamed noticeably, eat nothing at all for two or three days; then try a meal or two of very plain, unfermentable food, and after that fast a day or two, taking only liquids—fruit juices in the morning and vegetable juices in the afternoon, as much as you care for. Be sure to drink these juices slowly, allowing thorough salivation. As mentioned before, eat one kind of food only each mealtime.

Shall you eat fruits? In cases of gastritis, you would do well to avoid them for the time being, until your stomach is fairly well cleansed and healed, since gas is what we want to avoid, if possible. However, if you crave fruits particularly, you may eat them in small quantities. Sweet ferment is caused by the natural ether found in fruits when subjected to the digestive processes when these are not particularly strong. For the average healthy individual, fruits are practically non-fermentable.

Q. What is your opinion of the one-food meal?

A. Many cases of stomach and intestinal trouble are directly traceable to too complex mixtures, too generously partaken of. This is true of live foods as well as cooked foods, although in much smaller measure. If your stomach is in trouble and sends you pain or distress warning, do your share by giving it a rest. Eat nothing at all for a day, break your fast the next day, and fast again on the third and alternate days, for a week or two. On the days you eat, take one article of food at a time, with only a simple garnish if you think you need it. Each type of natural food, be it apples, lettuce, turnips, has in it, harmoniously combined, practically all of the elements needed to keep the human system in first-class condition. If your taste calls for a variety of foods, eat them at successive meals. You need not wait several hours—eat every hour or two if that is your desire. See that what you eat is thoroughly insalivated. Gas in the stomach is often caused by complex food mixtures. During the period of transition from cooked food to a mono diet of live fruits and vegetables, your taste may crave the more complex combinations. In such cases, and if you feel no discomfort after eating them, you may logically and safely do so. When, however, your stomach is sensitive or weak, you must by force of will limit your intake by the means described.

Q. Do you recommend a mono diet in case of stomach ulcers?

A. Put nothing whatever into your stomach but lemon juice with water, as sour as you can stand it—no solid food at all. Start with one ounce of lemon in a glass of water, and continue increasing the amount of lemon juice. Your stomach will call for more and more as time passes. What appears sour to you at first will seem scarcely noticeable later on. The lemon will neutralize the ulcer secretions and help to heal the ulcers themselves. Moreover, what is not used for this purpose will be carried into the rest of the body and will neutralize the excess acids there.

Then, by bowel injections, take the food you need to keep the body functioning. This should consist of cereal water, of unprocessed whole wheat or oats, prepared in the following manner: fill a two-quart fruit jar a third full of oatmeal, or whole wheat meal. Add water to within an inch or two of the top; put on the cap; shake; and let stand for a couple of hours or more. Then strain a cupful of this water and inject into the bowel morning, and again at noon, and at night. In this manner you will get enough nourishment to tide you along nicely, even to build flesh. The water should be of body temperature. I have seen bodies nourished in this manner for a period of well over three months, with no ill effects whatever either during or after. Besides the above, take an olive oil rub all over the body morning and night. The olive oil, too, will help nourish your body through absorption by way of the skin. Sunshine on the bare skin is also advisable; not too much at first if you aren't accustomed to it.

When you have an ulcerated stomach you must take great care not to irritate it by any solid food until the internal sores are healed. Irritation will make the condition progressively worse regardless of whether the food is cooked or uncooked.

Q. What causes soreness in the stomach and the alimentary canal? Would olive oil or orange juice help?

A. Suppose you try some warm peanut milk. Heat some water to blood temperature or five degrees higher. Stir in some finely ground raw Spanish peanuts, or, if you like them better, almonds, unbleached. Let it settle while maintaining the temperature, and drink. This drink has a good deal of natural oil in it and will aid in overcoming your soreness.

Q. After eating, I have an acid stomach. I have been obtaining relief by taking either milk of magnesia or bicarbonate of soda. Is this the proper thing to do?

A. No, it is not. These highly advertised substances are drugs, producing a poisonous effect upon the body as they are non-assimilable. Such mechanical alkalization will do for a while, but soon your stomach lining will become irritated, and ulcers, even cancer, will be upon you. Put your trust in fruits and vegetables. They are Nature's alkalizing agents. The longer you use them, the stronger and healthier you will be.

Q. Is it injurious to the stomach mucles to take a longer time than is necessary to evacuate? I have a habit of reading at this time.

A. Have you ever noticed a wild, unspoiled animal reading while it was evacuating?—in fact, doing anything else at the moment but just that? Conservation of energy is a great law of Nature. To conserve our forces, we must concentrate upon the task in hand, be it a conscious one or a reflex function of the body. To divide one's attention means to weaken the principal activity going on at the moment, which therefore becomes less effective and easy than it should be. Concentrate upon a single aim and purpose—that is a good precept. There is a tendency during evacuation to fix the attention sharply upon some detail or other. That is all right, but do not become engrossed in general activities like reading. No doubt this is an odd survival from the prehistoric days of the race, when it was necessary to watch for enemies, particularly at that semi-helpless time. Referring to your specific question, it is thought that prolapses are sometimes caused in part by such an unnatural practice as the one you mention.

STRENGTH AND WEAKNESS

Q. What is the cause of a weak feeling after one has been on raw food for a time?

A. You are full of phlegm, which the food is loosening. In the process of digestion, the stomach churns the food, works it from one side to another, and gets all the acids reduced until the whole has become an albuminous substance. This is perfectly normal. It is necessary to get the food thoroughly mixed there with the digestive fluids which neutralize the acid. As soon as the food is free from acid, the pylorus opens and the food material passes to the intestines. In the intestines are a multitude of little villi, tiny protuberances which absorb the nutriment from the food. Bile and the pancreatic juice are poured in to peptomize it. When the villi are clean, they will absorb the fine nourishment in live food. Yet we hear many who are beginning to live on this food say, "Doctor, I am weak. This food is no good. It doesn't give me any strength." The food is not to blame. These people have been eating dead food so long that they are brimful of catarrh, latent or otherwise. Its phlegm breaks from the nose into the pharynx, slips down into the stomach. From there it is carried to the upper bowel and entirely covers the villi with successive tough and almost impenetrable layers. Your food may be entirely correct and yet your villi will not be able to take hold of it to pass it on to the blood.

Before much nutriment can get through, you must break down this phlegm covering the villi. This sounds difficult, but it really is not. Eat an apple. Chew it, but not finely. Swallow when still quite coarse, be cause it will have to do a lot of grating and scraping on those villi before the phlegm will let loose. If you have no apples, do the same with a carrot—chew, and swallow the material when still coarse. These chunks will break up the phlegm. Should you have griping pains in the bowels after eating apples or carrots in this manner, rotate the hands over the bowels and they will be able to move. The movement will contain a phlegmy mass, the matter which has been loosened from the walls of the digestive tubes. Do this for some

time and you will begin to get some nourishment out
of your food.

Often, this weak feeling that is complained of is as
much nervous as physical. In such cases you can get
rid of the weak feeling temporarily by taking alternating hot and cold baths. Turn your shower twice hot and
twice cold, finishing on the cold. This relief, however,
will not be permanent, for the digestive tract will have
to be cleaned out. When the nerves are, like the villi,
in the process of being uncovered by the cleansing
action of the live food, they are apt to give you a
weak, or rather, "gone" feeling. This is not physical
at all, as I have said, and does not arise from a serious
shortage of nutriment. You are getting stronger all
the time, though you may not know it. Your emergency strength will be twice or three times as great as
it was before you started on the live food, and that is
the test. A change is taking place in your system, and
you must be patient enough to await the outcome ot
elimination.

Q. Please tell me what I can do to get stronger,
so that I can keep up my rather heavy physical work.
Raw food does not seem to nourish me very well.

A. Consult your tastebuds and see if you can find
something that will taste better than what you are eating. Such a food would be the one that is most nourishing to you at this time. Taste an assortment of different varieties of fruits, herbs, and roots. Try them
and find out for yourself—do not take anybody's word
for it. Have you tried the avocado? It is rich in fat.
Or why not tomatoes or cucumbers? Perhaps you

think tomatoes contain no nourishment, but there is just as much nourishment in tomatoes as anything that grows in Mother Earth, just as much as in the potato. I sometimes hear people say, "I like oranges very well but they are too dainty a food for me. I must have something more substantial for my work, say, a beefsteak or some eggs." Let me say that one half of a head of lettuce contains more food value than five pounds of beefsteak. The butcher will tell you there is no protein in lettuce. That is not true, for there is plenty of chlorophyll in lettuce, protein which will never cause protein poisoning. All flesh and dairy proteins, on the other hand, easily cause high protein poisoning.

Q. How can I best develop arm, leg, and stomach muscles? For two years I have lived exclusively on the raw food diet you recommend, and feel very well, but I lack muscular strength.

A. Nature gave us muscles not for show, but for use. The bank clerk presents a pathetic physical appearance; the farm hand often might model for a sculptor. Why? Because the farm hand has employed his muscles vigorously while the bank clerk has not. It is not necessary to be a farm laborer, however, to develop sturdy, efficient muscles. Fifteen minutes a day of well-balanced exercise will do marvels in as short a space of time as a month. The exercises should be simple at first, gradually becoming more complex as you become accustomed to the routine. You should exercise only a short time at first, gradually increasing the time. The benefit derived from exercise is depend-

ent largely upon the faithfulness with which you regard
the task of building your body. Allow no day to pass
without the exercises. Fifteen minutes a day for four
days will do splendid things for you. An hour every
four days is practically valueless, may even be detrimental, since it involves strain and overwork of the
muscles and ligaments.

What exercises should you do? That will depend
upon your individual needs. It may be that you require
special attention to various parts of the body, such as
legs, arms, chest, neck, stomach, etc. In such a case, you
must include not only general but also specific exercises designed to reach and stir that particular weak
part or organ. You will find in the public libraries any
number of books describing exercises in detail; there
are also exercise charts by authorities on health questions, and, finally, excellent courses in physical culture
which you may take by correspondence, if you wish.

SUNBATHING

Q. When taking sunbaths, should the body rest
directly upon the ground or should something be
spread to recline upon?

A. Do not be afraid to stand up and do some exercises while in the sunshine. Do not lie down if you
can help it, but keep moving about as in a state of
nature. There is too much dehydration of moisture
from the blood when you lie on the ground like a
prune or drying peach. As to ground covering, always
get as close contact with the soil as you reasonably
can. Go barefooted whenever you can. Even a partial
sunbath is much better than none.

Q. What is the best time of day for sunbathing, and how long should one indulge in it?

A. Do not take sunbaths, if you can help it, between eleven and two in this latitude. If no other time is available to you, however, it is all right, but the exposure should be shorter. Early forenoon or late afternoon is the ideal time. The duration of your sunbath should vary according to the amount of tan on your skin, the general condition of your health, and your desire for the sunshine. If your skin is perfectly white, do not venture out for more than about ten minutes for the first time. Lengthen the period gradually. If you are afflicted with certain diseases, do not take sunbaths at all, or short ones. In most cases, however, unless you are very weak, indeed, you can safely take sunbaths and you will benefit thereby. Sunbathing should always be done in the open, without window or curtain obstructions. Or, in the winter, you may raise the window of your room and enjoy the shaft of sunshine that comes in. Even if only for a few moments, it will stimulate you.

Q. Why does one sometimes feel weak after sunbathing?

A. You may have been in the sun too long. This will make itself felt even while you are out in it. There is, on the other hand, the natural relaxation that occurs when the body, made taut by the sun's rays, lets go. This latter feeling should be a pleasurable one, and is entirely normal.

SUNBURN

Q. Why do some people, especially those with light complexion, burn in the sun, while others tan?

A. Many people who are extremely light complexioned are so because of their ancestral living habits. They have for centuries kept away from the sun and air by reason of their clothes, buildings, and indoor occupations. Should they get into the sun, they would freckle, redden in color, but very seldom tan. The redness under the skin is really a sort of tan, for the darker color shuts off the sharp rays of the sun. Dark-complexioned people, on the other hand, will usually tan readily enough. Their skin is much thicker than that of blondes, and whereas fair-skinned individuals have much iron in the surface area of the skin, brunettes have little. As regards iron, freckles are composed largely of unassimilated deposits of iron. Light-complexioned people should be sure not to stay in the sun too long at any one time. Gradually they will find their skin turning a much darker color. This is especially true in sub-tropical and tropical climates. In a northern climate, where there is much cloudy and cool weather, they ought, on the other hand, to get as much direct sunshine on their entire body as they can. In this latter instance, if they consistently expose their bodies to the sun's rays, there will be no danger of painful sunburn. It is best to begin in childhood, with full sunbaths at least two or three times a week.

Q. How do you treat sunburn?

A. If the case is an old or chronic one, put on a

little sweet oil every day. If it is recent, try some lemon juice, straight; better yet, a mixture of sweet oil and lemon juice, making it quite strong. In all cases, it is wiser, to be sure, to prevent sunburn. Rub yourself with lemon juice before you go into the sun, and this will do the work. Orange juice also is beneficial.

To apply the lemon juice in the case of recent sunburn, dip a pad of absorbent cotton large enough to cover the area, into the juice. Put it on the sunburn, and leave it there all night. For the first few moments it will smart, but very soon complete relief will come. Avoid the use of drug store preparations, as these contain coal tar products in most cases, and are harmful rather than beneficial.

Q. Please tell me what is good for sunburn when blisters are forming with lots of pus.

A. Pus with your sunburn indicates bad blood condition. It is really a good thing you were sunburned, for thus you will get rid of some of your waste matter. Bathe the blisters with lemon juice or lemon water, and in the morning eat plenty of lemon with your food. Nothing neutralizes pus like lemon juice.

Q. Are those who eat natural food as subject to sunburn?

A. Certainly, unless they have a gradually-acquired coat of tan, as all live fooders should have. A coat of tan is simply a protection against excessive radiation from the sun. All things, however good, should be taken in moderation. The natural action of the skin in tanning shows the fundamental truth of this statement. Start your coat of tan early in the spring, when the sun rays are not yet strong. The early morning hours are the best. By the time summer arrives you will have acquired your tan so gradually and painlessly that when others are squirming with sunburn you will be cool and comfortable in even the hottest sunshine. There is a natural tendency for an under-irradiated, pale body to absorb all the sunshine it can in the shortest possible time. It craves this vitalizing force and hence gets an over-dose when exposed to the sun for all of a blazing summer's day on the beach. So even though you are not a salt pork eater (and these burn easily), observe here, too, the laws of life.

SUPERFLUOUS HAIR

Q. How would you permanently remove hair from the arms and legs otherwise than by the use of the electric needle?

A. Here is a possible way, not yet fully tried out; namely, the use of pine tar. When I was a youngster, my brother once threw a pine tar can at me. The skin was not broken, but a little dab of it struck me on the lip. No hair has ever grown on that spot since. Try a little of it in a limited area and see how it works. If it is satisfactory, try more elsewhere. It is disagreeable material to work with. In removing the pine tar, you must be prepared to see the hairs, with their rootlets, coming out also. That is why this method is supposed to be effective. Beauticians use this same principle.

Q. Can one remove superfluous hair without removing the roots?

A. I know of no effective method beside the one you mention. Yet you may bleach the hair by the use of peroxide, or, better, lemon juice. This latter will not work as quickly, perhaps, but it is more natural.

Do not worry too much about the unsightliness of such hair. After living for some considerable period on live food, and otherwise obeying Nature's laws, you will find that even if the hair has not stopped growing or disappeared of its own accord, at least it will have become harmonized with the rest of your personality and will no longer be felt a blot. For example, the sun itself will tend, over a period of time, particularly in women, to lighten the shade, which, together with the darkening of the skin, will help solve your problem.

SWELLINGS

Q. What shall I do for a swelling under my left breast? I weigh over one hundred seventy pounds.

A. Is it sore? If so, I would put on hot applications for half an hour, then a single cold one for a few minutes. Prepare a poultice of lemon pulp; keep it on over night, and in the morning the chances are that the swelling will be much reduced. Lemon is a splendid agent in reducing swellings. If the lump is not sore, continue with your live food 100 per cent, and the swelling will disappear.

Q. I am very much improved from the bladder inflammation after hot baths for a week. Thank you. I still have swollen fingers.

A. Take a dish sufficiently large so that when you fill it with lemon juice and put in your fingers, the liquid will entirely cover the swollen parts. But first put your fingers into hot water, as hot as bearable, and when the finger tips are red with blood, wipe dry, and swing through the air so that the coolness will cause the blood to recede. Then the lemon juice. Keep them there for some minutes. This will take down the swelling since lemon, besides being a strong disinfectant, is a mild astringent. Do this every night before going to bed.

Q. Every winter my feet become chapped and swell considerably, so that walking is painful. Is this a form of elimination? What shall I do for them?

A. Yes, it is a form of elimination. You might try walking on the dewy grass of a morning; also paddling about with them in mud. The one will tend to stimulate and strengthen; the other to draw out the poison and contract the tissue. All these natural practices are simple but efficient, as all Nature's remedies are.

SYPHILIS

Q. Can syphilis be cured? Will the introduction of mercury into the system have any influence on the time required?

A. Syphilis can be cured by natural methods. It sometimes takes a considerable period, and sometimes not, depending upon the individual—how far the disease has progressed and how much of the deadly mercury is in the system. The disease affects many organs, and each one must be treated locally. As to the mercury, we can get rid of it all in time. It matters not whether the syphilis is inherited or whether it is contracted by the patient. Natural food is an active force and will never rest until the system is entirely purified. I have learned that fresh coconut is one of the greatest eliminators in such cases. You will, in the course of time, suffer considerable local pain in the affected parts of the body. Whenever that happens, apply heat, either by hot water applications, hot water bottle, electric pad, or what not. The important thing is that blood be drawn to the region by the heat. The nerves will then be soothed and your pain will disappear. As the blood recedes, it will take with it much of the poisonous material collected there, including mercury.

The foods most suitable for you, besides the above-mentioned coconut, are: cantaloupe, tomatoes, watermelon, cucumbers. These latter four will flush your kidneys and thus aid elimination. A 100 per cent raw food diet is essential.

Wash yourself thoroughly every day. This is important. Take an alternate hot and cold shower bath each day to stimulate the action of the skin glands. The skin is as important an organ of elimination as the kidneys in many instances of high-pressure elimination. Take Epsom salt baths once or twice a week. Lemon-juice rubs are of value.

Q. Is the disease of syphilis widespread? Can it be contracted through the use of a public toilet?

A. It is much more widespread than is commonly

imagined. The rather loose morals of recent years, the so-called freer relationships particularly in regard to sex, have apparently widened its scope tremendously. Syphilis is a very serious disease, capable of transmission to innocent women and children. Hence it is important to be very careful, even fastidious, in the use of public conveniences such as toilets, not to mention sexual relationships. Often the disease is latent, not suspected even by the one who is the carrier. He may have contracted it earlier and, under the suppressive effect of mercury, consider himself cured, when as a matter of fact he has merely weakened his body to such an extent by the injections that it is not capable of throwing off the poisons of syphilis or kill the highly active germ involved in its progress. Cooked-fooders are constantly on the brink of a precipice as to all disease, including syphilis. Their bodies are full of phlegm, weak, and receptive to the inroads of disease bacteria. What a fertile ground these find here. Live fooders, on the other hand, offer little that is attractive to these minute organisms. They readily ward off all attacks because of the vigorous resistance of their bodily forces. The attacking army is routed before the battle fairly begins. If the enemy is already within your gates, lose no time in calling upon the most powerful, and indeed the only aid to renewed health; namely, natural, uncooked food.

Q. Is mercury treatment ever advisable for syphiletics?

A. Mercury is one of the most deadly of drugs, and is used for that reason, in the belief the body will,

when confronted with the new and even more potent
enemy, stop showing the symptoms which are typical
of the disease—syphilis. Notice that the symptoms are
merely suppressed and that the disease is by no means
cured. Its ravages are going on just as before, except
that the body no longer attempts to combat them.
Hence the patient suffers no pain or even discomfort
for the time being. When, however, the immediate
effect of the drug has been thrown off, the symptoms
will begin again. A negative Wasserman test will
turn to a positive, and a new dose of poison will be required, followed by another short period of assumed
cure. As time goes on, the body will become so saturated with the drug that a state of semi-paralysis is induced, not recognized as such by the patient, however.
He fancies himself cured, whereas it is merely that his
body forces have been reduced to the lowest possible
ebb. All the while the disease creeps on insidiously, and
perhaps after a period of years will begin to show its
might. By that time, it may have affected the spine,
even the brain. Natural living, not mercury, is the
wonder-worker.

Beware of skin ointments and cure-all patent medicines of any description. They usually contain mercury.
Some doctors claim to cure men's diseases, so called.
If these doctors are using natural methods, vegetable
and fruit products, and insist upon natural living, well
and good. If not, they are quacks, at the best, ignorant
seducers of the people.

TAPEWORMS

Q. How can I get rid of a tapeworm? What are the symptoms of its presence?

A. The most obvious symptoms are griping pains in the bowels and the discharge of sections of tapeworm in the bowel movements. A tapeworm can live only in the intestines of one who eats cooked food, particularly meat. A raw fooder would be an uneasy habitation for one, since it would soon become starved, shrivel up, and die. Tapeworms are scavengers which live on masses of waste material that collect in the bowels. Fat people are usually hospitable to them. Get rid of the foul waste in your body and you will have no trouble with worms. Anyone who eats live food will not be subject to the tapeworm, and if he had one before he changed his way of living, he will soon be rid of it. It is said that meats, particularly raw beef and pork, contain the tapeworm in embryo, which then proceeds to feed merrily and grow up, sometimes to huge size, in the body of the often unsuspecting victim.

There are two ways of eliminating the tapeworm: through starving or poisoning it. Live food kills it through starvation. Unthinking people take drugs for the purpose, but that, obviously, is a highly stupid procedure, since the patient as well as the tapeworm is poisoned thereby. One of the best simple remedies is to eat pumpkin seeds. Chew them well or grind them up previously. The next day take copious doses of castor oil. This will give the tapeworm its walking, rather, its gliding papers, for exit.

TEETH AND GUMS

Q. I have several silver and amalgam fillings in my teeth. Is it possible that the system can absorb mercury from the fillings, causing various ailments?

A. Mercury is derived from quicksilver. Quicksilver is not used in filling teeth. However, silver in the mouth forms an amalgam, which is a definite poison. So get these fillings out as quickly as you can. Replace them by porcelain or gold.

Q. I have been living on live foods for over a year. I have a small cavity in my front tooth. Can it be cured by exercises and right living?

A. Eat cabbage, carrots, and radish; also turnips, rutabagas, cauliflower, and celery—these noon and evening. Eat fruits in the morning. Do not eat acid fruits. The acid does no harm in itself but may get to the nerves of the tooth and pain you. The other foods mentioned will heal these nerves. If you have a cavity of any size, put some ordinary chewing gum in it. You can get the flavor and sugar out by kneading the gum under running water. Then watch your tooth fill itself. Several persons in this city have filled their teeth in that way. If your bloodstream is clean and you have never had syphilis or gonorrhea, teeth will do that.

Q. How can I improve my teeth? Would you recommend having them pulled and substituting a plate?

A. False teeth are well enough in their way, and

yet no substitute for the set Nature gave you. In my
practice I have noted some splendid instances of hollow teeth being refilled, of broken teeth growing back
to their full length, without other aid than natural
food. However, I find that this is not yet generally
believed. It may be necessary for grown-ups to live for
many years in Nature's way before they will be able
to accomplish this feat. Their bloodstream must first
be made vital. On the other hand, I know of men as
old as seventy-five who have grown another set of teeth.

A little girl nine years old was once brought to me.
Her broad front tooth had been broken in two by a
fall, leaving a two-thirds stump. She had been on an
ordinary cooked vegetable diet, plain and simple, yet
nothing really natural except an occasional raw apple
or raw onion. I said to the mother, "Why not put her
on a raw vegetable diet, raw cabbage, turnips, and
radishes? Do not include any fruit in the same meal."
She did so. In three months we noticed little icicle-
shaped points coming down from the broken end of
the tooth, about one-sixteenth of an inch long. They
could not be bitten on by the lower teeth because of
side tooth protection, and therefore they grew unhin-
dered. But when these grew longer and merged together, they lost their shape and little ribs began to
form. Before six months were up, the child had a
complete tooth. It was a little shorter than its mate,
a matter of a sixteenth of an inch or so. It was beautifully enameled, and no doubt in time became as long
as its neighbors.

Q. Is it necessary to have abscessed dead teeth extracted?

A. That depends upon how large the abscess is and of how long standing. If the abscess has been ulcerating so long that the nerve force is no longer able to come through to it, you had better have the tooth removed and the whole flesh cavity disinfected with lemon juice, so that it will heal up. But in most cases there is still plenty of healthy tissue around the tooth so that healing material can be brought in to where it is needed; perhaps even, in time, a new tooth will appear.

Q. Should dead teeth which have turned black after the removal or decay of the nerves, be pulled?

A. If your teeth are usable and do not annoy you or cause any pain, why pull them? They are better than any which the dentist can make for you, since they are firmly rooted. Of course, the color may not suit you, but that is of comparatively little importance if they are still serviceable. The teeth are never a primary source of infection. They merely collect the poisons which are afloat in the bloodstream. If your body is clean, there will be no abscesses, and if you have any when you begin, they will disappear. Lemon juice held in the mouth for some time, morning and evening, will, in contact with any hidden or obvious abscesses, help to reduce the swelling or inflammation and to drive the pus back into the bloodstream or mouth cavity for expulsion. Hot and cold water applications will also do much to relieve the temporary distress.

Q. If teeth are abscessed, should they be pulled?

A. If you have a boil or blister on any part of your body, you do not cut off that part but use more rational means to cure it. Why not cure an ulcer at the root of your tooth in the same way? All who have ulcers of the teeth should get a reading glass. In the morning, between ten and twelve, when the sun is shining brightly, locate the source of irritation on your gum. Move the tongue and cheek aside in such a manner so that you can focus the sunshine, by means of the reading glass, directly on the infection. Notice my directions, however. The sun shining through the glass will cross, and at the point where the rays meet, you can burn paper, cloth, wood, or flesh. You can even set fire to a man's hair in that manner. That is where the rays cross. But a short distance on either side of where they cross you have a beam of light one half the size of a dime. Here it will not burn, but will warm and penetrate the flesh. The reading glass should then be held so that not the point, but the wider diameter of the ray, comes in contact with the flesh; then there will be no burning but helpful irradiation. Do this every morning for about ten minutes, and continue until results are apparent, which will be quite soon. Lemon juice, or the pulp of a lemon, will also soak in. Lemon is a deadly enemy to pus or degenerate tissue of any kind. Hot water applications, alternating with cold, or a sip of hot water in the mouth, will also aid.

Q. Does lemon shrink the gum from around the teeth?

A. Lemon juice cures pyorrhea; it does not shrivel or shrink the gums but, rather, brings them back to a normal condition. If the gums are inflamed with pus, it might appear to do so, but in time the gums will become firm again.

Q. Is there a cure for pyorrhea? I am a raw fooder.

A. Lemon is a great remedy for pyorrhea. Roll a lemon soft, cut it crosswise, squeeze part of the juice out, and cut lengthwise into little strips one-half an inch wide. These will come to a point at the end. Put one of these strips into the mouth, your finger on it, and use like a brush: rub gently back and forth across the gums. You may want to use several of these for one cleansing. This is the cleanest and most antiseptic brush you can get. Take a mouthful of the juice, rinse the oral cavity with it. It will help get your gums hardened. The rest of your pressed-out juice you may dilute with some water and drink. There is much uric acid in your system. For this, eat natural foods 100 per cent. Try a little horseradish once a day, a tablespoonful at evening with a few flaked peanuts. Horseradish is a good antiseptic. Take Epsom salt baths once a week. This is for the purpose of opening the pores so that the salts will be able to draw out the poisons. Remember to keep the water at blood heat and to rub off the slime from your body at the end of every ten-minute immersion, the bath consisting of as many of these periods as is needed to cleanse your blood for the time being. A cold dash at the conclusion of the whole is stimulating.

Q. Would it not be possible to cure pyorrhea by some of the astringent toothpastes now on the market especially advertised for that purpose?

A. These toothpastes are composed of astringent drugs and are not in the remotest sense natural products. These drugs will find their way, at least in part, to the alimentary canal and then the bloodstream. Drugs are poisons and should never be used. Since they must be thrown out sooner or later by the body, the eliminative organs become overtaxed and weakened. Sometimes when these artificial preparations are used, the gum bleeding stops and you think you are cured. Hence the testimonials in advertisements. The effect is always temporary, however, and sooner or later the pyorrhea will come back more virulent than ever when the immediate effect of the drug has passed off. Neither doctors nor dentists can accomplish a cure when they disregard natural laws, and neither can you.

Q. How can you relieve a painful swollen gum caused by a crowned tooth pressing down too far?

A. Roll a lemon; cut it in half, and slice out a piece large enough to put between the cheek and the teeth at the place of infection. Leave it there until all the juice is out of it. Several hours later try another piece. Keep this up until the swelling is gone. If the dentistry is at fault, revisit your dentist and have it corrected.

Q. I have a painful tooth with a considerable cavity in it. Can I do anything to relieve it?

A. If you want to have it filled, have the dentist use porcelain or gold, and avoid corrosive drugs in the process of filling. If you prefer to wait upon the slower filling-in by the hand of Nature, put in a piece of chewing gum from which the sugar and flavor have been removed by kneading under a faucet. Press well into the cavity. It will remain there nicely if in not too exposed a position. Try hot and cold applications also.

Q. For teeth and gums too sore for raw foods, would you recommend foods softened by steaming or cooking?

A. No. There are shredders on the market which reduce raw vegetables to a feathery consistency so that they can be assimilated with scarcely any chewing. They should be insalivated thoroughly in the mouth, however, before swallowing. Fruits like persimmons, tomatoes, avocados, peaches, plums, etc., can be eaten, pulp and all, with little chewing. If you have any difficulty, mash them with a fork. Berries, too, can be eaten in this manner. Then you may, if you care to, drink vegetable and fruit juices, unheated and uncanned, and direct from the squeezer. These latter are very fine. Your system needs bulk, however, and you should eat as much of the natural fruit or vegetable as you can.

Q. I am having trouble with my crowned teeth. Does that indicate the body is trying to throw off poisons? What can be done about it?

A. The system is evidently eliminating a good deal of acid, and in doing so is loosening the fillings and the crowns. Do not be alarmed—the acid will soon b.: out of your system. Save the loosened crowns until the acid has disappeared. You can make a litmus paper test yourself: blue litmus paper under the tongue, if it does not change color, indicates an alkaline condition. You may then have the crowns put back on again. They will stay there without any further trouble.

Q. Tartar deposits accumulate on my teeth. Should I have them removed by a dentist? The tartar goes up under the gums.

A. Even if you should have the deposits removed, in a short time they would accumulate again. Tartar means that your diet is wrong; the acid condition of your system makes its appearance inevitable. As soon as you get your body completely alkalized, the tartar will disappear permanently. Meanwhile, apply lemon juice, using a soft cloth, or rub teeth and gums with some lemon pulp.

Q. Do you advise periodic visits to a dentist?

A. If your technique of living is correct, you need not worry about visits to the dentist. Even if cavities are already started, they will grow no larger. In fact, they may fill up with enamel as time goes on. Teeth fed by a healthy bloodstream will never decay.

TOBACCO

Q. Is smoking injurious?
A. The so-called pleasure derived from smoking is due to the absorption of nicotine into the body by

way of the lungs and stomach, particularly the former. It is very deadly poison. One drop will kill a cat. Even a whiff of nicotine will kill smaller animals. Nicotine is a compound of three elements—carbon, hydrogen, and nitrogen — 10 parts, 14 parts, and 2 parts, respectively. Chemists know what a poisonous substance this combination is. When you once have acquired this noxious habit, you are loathe to give it up—as long as you remain living on the food which gives you that craving, predisposed your system toward its use. But begin living a natural, raw-food life, and soon you will become so sensitive to nicotine poisoning that, not to mention you yourself smoking, you will not be able to remain in a room where there is smoking going on, so offensive will it be.

Q. I am twenty-five years old and smoke a pipe. I do not seem to be able to quit it. Can you tell me how?

A. When you once make up your mind to stick to natural living, your main troubles will be over. In a short time you will not be able to smoke, no matter what the outside incentive. Your body will have become cleansed sufficiently, will have thrown off enough of the nicotine, to make you very susceptible to even minute doses of the drug. Natural foods cure the worst cases of addiction to tobacco. To be sure, habitual users will go along for some time without seeming to feel any good effects. Meat-eating in particular seems to have an irritating influence upon the human organism, which then lends itself easily to the narcotic effects of tobacco, liquor, and other drugs. All these habit-forming substances seem to come in each other's train. Eat cooked foods and you will soon feel a craving for meat, pastries, dairy products, and all the foodless foods imaginable. This in turn makes it easy for tobacco to win a place. Then comes alcohol. Finally, when these no longer give the required jolt to the nervous system, there are available still more powerful drugs. They are a witch's ring, dancing hand in hand around the destruction of the human body and mind. "Give the devil a finger and he will take your whole hand," is an old saying. You cannot shake hands with God and the devil at the same time. To live on live food, together with attention to fresh air, sun-shine, bathing, conservation of energy, and exercise, means a new life entirely different and distinct from the old. The eating of cooked food lies at the very heart of our modern corruption. Eliminate that, and you will have struck at the source of physical and moral decay.

Q. Are there cigarettes which do not harm the nerves?

A. It is interesting to note that in Russia a nicotine-less tobacco has been propagated and is about to be put into production on a large scale. The ill effects of tobacco are recognized by Russian scientists, as the government there, I understand, encourages the use, meanwhile, of the partially denicotinized leaf. It is well known that the fully denicotinized product does not satisfy the user, and very likely this nicotine-free plant will be unpopular commercially and will not be bought as long as the other is available.

You may find cigarettes which are made of tobacco with either part of their nicotine content removed, or else made of so-called "mild" leaf. In modern cigarette advertising, the so-called "mild" cigarettes may be smoked all day long without a too immediately tangible effect. The harsher tobaccos would, on the other hand, literally rip the nervous system to pieces in comparatively short order. The only difference between these and the milder ones is that the latter are more deliberate in producing the same effect. Smoke enough of the mild cigarettes, or smoke them long enough in point of time, and your body will be as thoroughly poisoned as it can be this side of death.

Q. Is it not true that smoking tends to quiet the nerves?

A. So it does, but it is the quiet of death. Take enough of this nicotine and your nerves will be stilled forever. A narcotic effect is produced, combined with a recently discovered stimulating effect upon the adrenal glands. The jangling nerves are put into a lethargy, at the same time animal pugnacity is stirred up by the jolt given the glands. "What could be finer!" you say. "I feel refreshed and invigorated." You will notice, however, unfortunately, a more than corresponding feeling of lassitude, of dejection, shortly after. This means that the adrenals are now functioning below normal, after the period of over-exertion during which they were unnaturally stimulated. Also, the body is now beginning to throw off the nicotine through the regular channels. The nerves have recovered from their semi-paralysis and jangle worse than

ever. What then could be more refreshing and invigorating than a second cigarette? This time, however,
you feel less refreshed, and the depression is slightly
worse. Each time you smoke you will find the habit
getting more firmly ingrained. Larger and larger doses
will be required to satisfy you. Liquor and violent
drugs may follow in logical order.

Q. Is smoking more injurious to women than to
men?

A. Yes, because of the fact that women, biologi-
cally, are delicately built. Their tissues are more per-
meable by poisons, more easily damaged than those of
men. Their sex organs, particularly, are subject to
atrophy by nicotine. As regards childbearing, even
newspapers bring reports of children who, through
the mothers' breasts, have consumed enough nicotine to
become addicts at that pathetically tender age. Other
reports speak of children who become violently ill
after partaking of their mothers' milk. Whenever a
mother smokes, an appreciable percentage of nicotine
is found in the milk. In many cases, however, inability
to nurse is directly traceable to smoking. The mammary glands are dried up. Furthermore, in conclusion,
just how romantic is a tobacco-scented kiss, just how
enticing to the male? A woman naturally wishes to be
alluring and attractive to the opposite sex, so why
should she deliberately reduce her charm by vicious
habits? Then we must consider the effect of example
upon the growing child. What child will feel con-
strained to keep away from tobacco when it sees its

mother smoking? All this does not excuse men, of course.

Q. My young son, through association with his fellow students at high school, has acquired the smoking habit. How should I go about getting him to break it?

A. The most important thing is to have a heart-to-heart talk with him about the effects of tobacco upon the human system. Show how nicotine reduces the efficiency of the muscles and the glands, the clearness of thought. Impress upon him that no real man will ever use tobacco unless he is ignorant of its true nature, that only weaklings with insufficient strength to face the facts of life will seek the support of a narcotic such as tobacco. The best way for him to break the habit is to break it at once and completely. If he were living on an alkaline diet; that is, on live food, the odor and taste of tobacco would be distasteful to him. Therefore, it should not be difficult.

TONSILS

Q. Practically all doctors tell people they must have their tonsils removed. Do you think they must?

A. The tonsils are the sentinels that guard the stomach from unnatural foods. When your tastebuds or teeth discover something that should not go down into the stomach, your tonsils prevent you from swallowing it. The tonsils also are signal governors; they give signals to the thyroid gland, stimulating it to give out a magnetic influence which aids in the proper digestion of certain food. When removed, there will be a sense of distinct loss; for example, lacking them, you can never be a good singer. So do not think Nature made a mistake in placing them where she did. We should try to aid and not try to improve upon her work.

Q. What is the best remedy for bad tonsils?

A. First, get rid of your disease-building habits: cooked food eating; inactive muscles and mind; insufficient sleep, fresh air, and sunshine; wasting vital energies. Begin living according to the laws of Nature. Specifically, in the way of remedy, put hot and cold applications on the neck, alternating, and ending with a cold. Then, when plenty of blood has been collected in the neck region, do some neck exercises, so that the blood will be absorbed into the muscles.

Diseased tonsils are usually swollen. This is called "tonsilitis." There is nothing that will reduce the swelling more quickly than the juices and fumes of certain fruits. Several apples, for example, eaten each night on retiring lying flat on the back in bed, will bathe the tonsils in their alkaline fluid and quickly reduce them to normalcy. If your teeth are not good, grind the apples into a mash. Swollen tonsils often have been aided by eating daily a small handful of dried olives, which are rich in potassium.

Q. Will tonsils, once removed, ever grow back in again?

A. Sometimes they do, particularly when the person lives on live food and is in good physical condition. It depends somewhat on how the operation was performed. If they were not cut down too deeply, the

chances for their reappearance are better than otherwise. I have seen several cases of an entirely new set
of tonsils being grown after an operation.

TUBERCULOSIS OF THE BONES

Q. Can tuberculosis of the bone be cured? If so,
how long should it take? I have in mind a child fourteen years of age with tuberculosis of the leg bone.

A. Natural foods can reconstruct the entire body,
bone and flesh and nerve. If a child of that age lives
100 per cent on this food, a cure may require from
three to five years. With an older person, it would
take longer. As bone is a dense material, the afflicted
parts should also have special treatments to hasten
local elimination and prepare for rebuilding. I mean
very hot water applications, with violet ray or sunshine and exercise in connection. These things are all
very essential.

The best kind of food to rebuild bone is found in
turnips, cabbage, rutabaga, and carrots; also, un-
roasted peanuts. The patient should have one entire
meal of this bone-building material every day. In the
morning let him eat fruits, herb vegetables at noon,
roots at night. He may have raw peanuts with his
vegetables and roots, preferably flaked. The vegetables
and roots should be served tastily if the child is not
accustomed to them in their natural state. However,
the dressings should be very simple—olive oil, and
perhaps a little lemon juice. Honey also is a tasty and
wholesome addition to salads.

The predisposition of tuberculosis of the bones is very often hereditary, but no one who lives naturally need fear. Plenty of sunshine is especially essential, together with the bone-building foods mentioned, as well as others that contain plenty of calcium, as for instance oranges, and certain varieties of grapes. Exercise in the fresh air is also invaluable.

TUBERCULOSIS OF THE LUNGS

Q. Please tell a man who has had t. b. for several years if there is any hope. He is now so weak that he cannot get up from bed.

A. Certainly there is hope. As long as there is life there is hope, but get busy. If his condition is such, he must be given an Epsom salts bath three times a day (in less severe cases once a day). Put two pounds of Epsom salts into a tubful of blood-warm water. These baths will cleanse the skin pores of phlegm. He will at once feel better because the blood, not being able to get sufficient air from the lungs, will get some oxygen through the pores of the skin cleansed in this manner. The watchword is "Wash, wash, wash." Tuberculosis is a filthy job; the patient is full of phlegm, so both plain water and Epsom salt baths are required. Regarding the effect of air on the skin, as little clothing as possible should be worn so as to stimulate the pores to activity. Much waste matter goes out every day by that medium, even under normal conditions. Sunbaths, too, stimulate the skin and strengthen the body. These latter, however, should be taken in moderation, especially at first. So much for the various types of baths.

Now a few words about food: watercress and mustard greens are splendid for tubercular patients because of their stimulative effect on the kidneys. Peaches, too, are splendid. They contain natural prussic acid. (This is not the inorganic and deadly form, but a very beneficial one. Inorganic prussic acid kills, but natural, organic prussic acid is of direct value to the body.) The peaches should not be peeled. Nectarines and apricots also belong to the peach family. The patient should get plenty of fruit juices, and if he cannot eat peaches as they are, he should have the extracted juice. Uncooked pumpkin is valuable also, for it is rich is phosphorous, live phosphorous, not the kind you get in the drug store, or the match box. The banana is an anti-tubercular food. It must be ripe; that is, the skin must be speckled and the tip yellow before eating. Some iron, as in the form of lettuce, is essential; some flaked nuts also, perhaps walnuts or almonds. Honey cuts phlegm, and should be used freely in cases of tuberculosis, either with the food or separately. Red cherries fit right into the picture at this point also. Evenings, the sufferer should have carrots if he likes them, nicely shredded, with a simple dressing, or, better, plain. Above all, no dairy products should ever be used. These are among the worst phlegm producers. In the average hospital, the tuberculosis patient is crammed with this death-dealing stuff. If he gets well, it is in spite of and not because of the food. Ham and eggs, red meat, and all unnatural food must be avoided at the pain of losing the fight for life.

Q. I have tuberculosis of over a year's standing. Now I am in the second stages. Please tell me how to cure it.

A. Tuberculosis is a catarrhal disease in which a germ feeds on the waste matter in the body. Stop eating the foods which gave you this disease, and start getting fresh air and sunshine, together with natural, wholesome raw foods. Eat the fruits you like best, although certain ones have more value for you than others at present. There is no better food remedy than the peach family. After each morning meal of these, take three ounces of flaked almonds, pignolias, or walnuts. If the fresh peaches are out of season, you may soak the sundried, unsulphured variety in water until soft. Drink the water if not entirely absorbed. You may use honey to sweeten. At noon, try some green herbs: lettuce, watercress, spinach, or cabbage, according to taste. In the evening: carrots are good unless you are sick in bed, in which case have only the juice.

Another important item—fresh air. Sleep out of doors, under the sky, where there is a continuous circulation of air. Pay no attention to those who say it is damp, or cold. Put on more blankets; also, eat warming foods. If you want to get your blood moving, you should eat garlic, peppers, radishes, watercress, mustard greens. That is the kind of heat you want, the living fire that grows in plants. When you once get this natural fire into the blood, you won't complain about the cold. You will thereby also get up a form of combustion in the system to destroy the phlegm that the t. b. germs are living on.

Keep on in this way for some months. Perhaps you will arrive at a beneficial crisis in about nine months or a year. At this time, you will throw up phlegm by the cupful. It will have gathered in the crevices of the lungs, and some day up it will come, and the next day too, and the day following. You will wonder at it. Then, never lie on your back but on your face, so that your tongue will fall forward and you will not choke. Do not worry, because Nature lubricates this exit with a fine serum in order that, when ready, the poisons may come out easily.

Throughout this year, take Epsom salt baths at least once a day. When your skin gets slimy, sponge it off. Then try it again, and so on, until no more phlegm exudes for the time being. Finish up with a cold sponge.

Rest and sunshine will do their part to heal you. Go to bed at sunset; avoid excitement. Take sunbaths between nine and eleven in the morning, while exercising, not lying down. These sunbaths should be nude. Let the sun shine on every part of your body, particularly the back and the crotch.

Q. When a person has tuberculosis so badly that he spits and vomits blood, is there any hope?

A. A tubercular case with blood hemorrhages is more hopeful than one without. Cases complicated with anaemia or low blood pressure are the more dangerous, as a hemorrhage from the lungs will clean out waste matter. We must try to stop the hemorrhages by natural means, nevertheless, but let us not be discouraged because of them. Tuberculosis in the more advanced stages is incurable as long as you eat cooked food, but is an easy thing to cure by natural methods.

Q. What is meant by this: occupational pulmonary tuberculosis, incipient stage?

A. It means that the lung disease which has just taken hold is caused by an unhealthful occupation or profession. It may be mining, bookkeeping, painting, working in a cotton mill, metal polishing, and others. It means too little live food, fresh air, sunshine, exercise, and rest. I advise such people to find themselves a new occupation, one, if possible, which keeps them out of doors. Much, however, can be accomplished by spending all your time outside of working hours in the open air. Sleep, eat, and play in the out-of-doors.

Q. Just what part does a dry climate play in the treatment of pulmonary tuberculosis?

A. Dryness may be of benefit, but of more importance is temperature. The patient should live in a region where it is possible to be out of doors the year 'round—sleep, eat, and play out of doors. Mild cases will be benefited immensely by sunshine, but those far advanced in the disease should not be exposed until they are stronger. Fresh air, natural food, plenty of rest, are of the utmost importance. If you can, in addition, get a dry climate, well and good, but a dry climate alone is not sufficient.

Q. Does sexual over-indulgence help to bring about tuberculosis?

A. Excess of any kind, long continued, helps bring about this dread disease, provided there is a tendency toward it. Sexual over-indulgence is particularly to be avoided since it depletes the body of the fluids essential to life and vigorous activity.

Q. Is it dangerous to live with a tubercular patient who is constantly coughing up disease-laden phlegm?

A. You need not be afraid unless you yourself are living in such a manner that the tuberculosis germ will find an hospitable breeding ground in your body. A healthy person will repel the germs easily. These germs are in the air and all about you, seeking human bodies full of poisons, where they may act as scavengers. If you are clean within and without, you may rid your mind of all such fears.

TUMORS

Q. Can a tumor of the stomach be cured, and how?

A. First you must stop eating. When the stomach is weak or diseased, you must never give it work to do. Take nourishment by way of the rectum, by oil rubs, and breathing of wholesome fresh air. The only food you should put into your stomach is that which tends to disintegrate the tumor. By this I mean lemon juice, perhaps half a tablespoonful in a little water twice a day. It will take from three to six weeks to cure a case, according to the size of the tumor.

Q. What diet is indicated for one who is suffering from a tumor in the stomach?

A. Only lemon juice is to be taken directly into the stomach. Feed yourself by way of bowel injections until your stomach is well, because when you have a tumor it must first be disintegrated and absorbed before you eat any food in the usual manner. Do not be alarmed about starving because you are likely rather to gain weight. The liquid bowel food should be prepared in the following manner: fill a jar half full of wholewheat or oat meal, add water to the top. Let it stand over night, and the next morning drain off a cupful of the liquid, straining out the coarse material. Heat to body temperature and inject through a regular syringe by way of the rectum. The bowels will absorb the nutriment in this liquid while the stomach is convalescent. Take this injection twice a day. Also, rub yourself down morning and evening with olive oil. Allow the oil to penetrate into the body by means of the pores. In other words, do not rub off the excess oil at once or put on your clothes; give yourself a half-hour air bath. By that time the bloodstream will have absorbed a great deal of the nutriment in the oil and then you may cleanse your body in preparation for dressing. Take slow, deep breaths of fresh air every day, preferably in connection with exercises. You are likely, for a time, to have running bowels, but do not worry—the stomach must have a rest, and, besides, you will have to get rid of much phlegmy material in this way. Everything will quite soon be restored to normalcy, and when it is, you will commence to get

hungry. Then eat a little food. If there is any indica·
tion of pain in the stomach, stop, and resume your oil
rubs, etc., until the tumor is completely gone. If there
is no pain, you make take moderate quantities of food
in the normal manner.

Q. What are the foods you recommend for the
elimination of a tumorous condition?

A. You need eliminative foods—all fruits are eliminative. If you are in a hurry to eliminate, eat fruits
in the morning and at noon. In the evening eat, preferably, root vegetables, or, if you choose, herbal vegetables. When you have been on raw food for six
months, commence to alternate your foods—one day
liquids and one day solids, for a week or two; or, considerably more rigorous, two days liquids and one day
solids. This is in the nature of a fast, and will get you
really hungry, and hunger is a first-rate tonic in itself.
Do not, however, go long periods without eating; you
are simply consuming your own flesh and nervous tissue thereby. You need not, of course, swerve from the
regular live food diet perscribed by me—the fruit,
herb, root balanced diet—but it will take longer for
you to get well.

Q. Would it not be advisable to have a tumor removed by surgical operation even though one lives
on live food?

A. Operations cost money and pain. You are filled
full of ether and other dopes, and besides, you are
risking your life. Scar tissue left by operations is a
distinct hindrance to normal functioning of the organs.

Moreover, why throw away your money and put your life in the balance when Nature will remove the obnoxious growth quickly, painlessly, and safely? By living a natural life, you are getting at the heart of the trouble. The tumor is a symptom, the sign of an attempt by the body to get rid of some of the excess waste matter. Remove the cause and you remove the tumor.

Q. Is it possible to get rid of a wen on the head? If so, please state how.

A. A wen is a tumor with a fatty substance in it. In this location it is perfectly harmless to have it cut out if the surgeon understands his job. The scalp being quiet tough and remote from the central currents of blood flow, removal by purely natural means may take rather too long for the patience of most of us. Use hot and cold applications if you prefer the strictly natural methods; sunshine every day, and perhaps its concentration by means of a reading glass; vigorous massage with the finger tips; as well as copious washing. All these are essential for the non-surgical reduction and elimination of the wen.

ULCERS

Q. What is your treatment for ulcers?

A. The best remedy for an ulcer, whether it be boil, carbuncle, a running sore, or internal ulcer, is to destroy the pus which it secretes and which has brought it about. To do this we use a harmless remedy, called lemon juice. Mix water and lemon quite strong to

taste. If the trouble is in the stomach, sip the lemon
juice down. If it is an open sore, take a syringe or
absorbent cotton, and apply. It will sting you for a bit
but will destroy the phlegmy matter. If you keep it up,
the healing process will soon take care of your sores.
Be sure you eat foods which cool your blood, such as
fruits that are not too sweet.

Q. A young girl twenty-one years old suffers pains
in the stomach after eating. There is doubt whether
it is ulcers or nervous indigestion. Please state the difference between the two.

A. If there are ulcers, there will be a sharp pain
like pin pricks or the cut of a knife. When there is
vomiting in connection, with pus in it, you have a
sure sign of ulcers. If this should be the case, taking
food into the stomach is to be strictly avoided, excepting only the juice of half a lemon with water,
three times a day. For nourishment, use rectal injections of cereal water, lukewarm, a cupful three times
a day. Put ground whole wheat or oats in a jar, soak
overnight, with plenty of water to spare. In the morning, drain off, strain through cheesecloth, heat, and
inject. An ordinary syringe may be used. Rub your
body with olive oil daily. Nourishment may thus be
absorbed through the skin also. Keep up this treatment
until you begin to get really hungry, which may be a
matter of weeks. The sharp pains will have disappeared by this time. Then consult your tastebuds as to
the food you would like. It may be lettuce, or an apple, or what not. Lettuce is one of the tenderest of
herbs, and perhaps the best to break a fast on. Eat just

a little at first, experimentally. If the results are good, you may have some more. If not, keep up the treatment for a while longer. You may wish to try the alternate-day fast treatment: only liquids one day, and solids the next. This is of course only for the convalescent stage, when your stomach does not refuse food entirely but still seems comparatively weak.

Q. What is the cause of ulcers?

A. The eating of cooked foods, particularly highly spiced ones. A chronic irritation is set up in the most exposed portion of the stomach. This refers to stomach ulcers. In other parts of the body, they may be due to an old wound which will not heal because of the toxic condition of the blood, or some other sore which becomes a channel of elimination for toxic wastes, so pressed is the body for allies in its fight with accumulated wastes within. Externally, too, atmospheric germs are an irritative influence in such spots. There are so-called ulcers which are merely latent and do not have the outward appearance of sores.

UNDERWEIGHT

Q. What food would be advised for a person who wants to gain weight?

A. First, I advise you to get rid of all the waste matter in your system. To do so, you will have to lose a good deal of weight. The old, half-dead tissue, saturated with poisons, must make way for new, live tissue, built up from natural food. That may take considerable time and patience, but when you once have no more waste matter in your body, you will invariably gain weight until you reach normal. Nature may seem to work too slowly to satisfy you, but just as soon as your body is thoroughly clean, you will gain weight. It is just a matter of getting the human organism into proper condition. Until such a time, let your tastebuds guide you toward the more eliminative foods.

Q. When one is striving to gain weight, is it possible to overeat on raw food?

A. Yes, you can overeat on natural as well as unnatural foods. When you overeat on cooked foods, you may have distress for several days. When you overeat on natural foods, there will be mostly only a feeling of uncomfortable fullness, and this will pass in the course of a couple of hours. But overeating is overeating, and a good rule to follow is to eat until you are satisfied, until your stomach sends the signal which means enough, and not too much. As far as weight is concerned, eating a small quantity that is relished and fully absorbed will do you more good than a large amount that is not.

Q. I have been on a 100 per cent raw food diet sixty days. Have lost thirty pounds, and am still losing. Am now twenty-five pounds underweight. What do you advise?

A. Keep right on until you get all the waste matter out of your system. You will never be really well until that time arrives. Do not be afraid about losing too much weight or strength. Nature will take care of that. Elimination can be slowed down by eating less juicy fruits and more herbs and roots.

Q. For one who is underweight, what specific foods would you prescribe?

A. First, you must assist digestion. Olives are an aid to digestion because they are rich in potassium. This element helps to break up the food cells without destroying the life. These are fat-producing foods in their most easily digested form: almond butter, raw peanut butter, flaked pecans and pignolias, coconut milk, bananas, oatmeal, and the like. All are in the raw food dietary. You may also want to add some of the herbs, like okra (gumbo) ; also raw soups that contain oil; flaxseed bread; or olive bread. Never over-eat if you can help it—you waste too much energy and have none left for either rebuilding your body or for activity in your daily occupation. Weakness, often present when eliminating, is sometimes due to improper use of bodily forces. When you eat enormous quantities of food, a great deal of energy is required and is hence not available for other purposes.

Q. Is it true that exercise helps build weight?

A. A peculiar fact about live food is that, if you lounge about all day, you will not pick up flesh. If, on the other hand, you will pitch in and go to work, exercise your muscles thoroughly each day, you will gain plenty of poundage and hard muscle, too, not fat. When you work, your muscles absorb the blood, which brings building material. If there is a scanty supply of blood, there can be only scanty building. This exercise should be in the sunshine, if possible. You need not work eight hours a day, physically, but your muscles should show signs of being tired at the end. Mere free arm exercises are not sufficient as a rule— the muscles must feel weight resistance, preferably progressively increasing, for real muscle building. You can work either in the garden, saw wood, or manipulate dumbbells or other gymnastic apparatus. If you have nothing else, heavy stones tossed about will serve the purpose. Too much physical activity, however, is just as bad as too little, and this applies to mental activity as well, and especially while eliminating. When you are tired, stop. There are work tastebuds as well as food tastebuds.

Q. Do dairy products increase bodily weight?

A. A man of my acquaintance lets his children run around nude in the sun. They live on raw food, but do not look very plump. His neighbor's children are fed on milk, bread and butter, cheese, eggs, and look as though they weigh twice as much. Unfortunately, however, they are always sick, like other children who live on cooked food and dairy products. One day both sets of children were weighed. It was found that the big, fat girls did not weigh any more than his little children did. These were not large in frame, but were packed with hard, mineral-rich flesh. All this was aside from the fact that they were continuously bright and active, never ill.

The so-called standard weights set up by medical men as normal are based on the wrong principle of living. When you live according to Nature, the body is never bulky, and neither is it scrawny—it will be beautifully rounded, lithe, and continuously active. Heaviness means non-activity—Nature-weight means things accomplished, and happiness, for both child and adult. So ignore weighing machines and the opinions of persons not versed in the new way of living.

VACCINATION

Q. Do you advise vaccination?

A. Certainly not. Vaccine, or lymph virus, is nothing but pus, and pus should be avoided, not sought after. We should do all we can to prevent legislatures from making laws that will force us to be innoculated when healthy or at any other time. Fortunately, some states do not make vaccination compulsory.

Many mothers cannot nurse their babies. What brought this condition about? Oftentimes, vaccination. It dries up the natural fluids in women. It is an unnatural practice and should be avoided at all costs. Laws, of course, are laws, and have to be obeyed, yet we should do everything in our power to prevent their passage, or work for repeal.

The heart is often affected by this unnatural operation, and the worst of it is that we do not suspect that the most important of our organs has been thus weakened. Chronic heart disease is on the increase, largely for this reason.

Q. What about compulsory vaccination? Is there anything we can do to neutralize the harmful effect of the virus?

A. Immediately after the injection, be prepared with a bottle of lemon juice; better yet, whole lemons. Cut one in half, put over the spot where you have been vaccinated, and leave there for about half an hour. Then wash off with warm water. Lemon will kill the worst poison known.

Q. Is it true that vaccination is unlawful in Europe?

A. England has tabooed vaccination. The vaccination delirium began in England, and it is also the first nation to make vaccination a criminal offense. It has learned its lesson in the late war. Italy has done the same. When are we Americans, supposed to be the most enlightened people in the world, going to stop innoculating healthy persons with pus from sick animals? Injecting anything into the blood is the most unnatural of procedures. Nothing should ever be taken into the system except through the channels provided by the body.

At the present time high medical opinion has stated that vaccination emphatically does not prevent disease, that there is just as much smallpox, for instance, among those who are vaccinated, as among those who are not. Vaccinations for colds, skin diseases, and other common ailments, are an important part of the medical racket in our day. The lure of gold lies at the bottom of these specious attempts to improve our health.

Q. Has not yellow fever been stamped out by vaccination?

A. No. Improved drainage, house screens, and like preventive measures, are responsible. The injection of pus into a system itself overloaded with phlegm, has never yet, nor ever will, prevent or cure any disease. In fact, no honest person will ever claim that disease is prevented: just the contrary—the disease is imparted. Only a slight case, however, is hoped for. But who will guarantee it? Many deaths actually due to vaccine and its ensuant disease, are ascribed hypocritically to various other causes. Now and then reports of an epidemic of deaths will leak out, even into our newspapers. These epidemics are especially common among children.

VARICOSE VEINS

Q. Is there any cure for varicose veins?

A. Varicose veins are enlarged veins, since the valves have become ruptured. These valves, four inches apart, then can no longer control the blood supply as they should, but allow the veins to become chronically enlarged. As this is the reason for the condition, you must again close these valves. How can this be done?

Live on natural foods for at least six months. This will eliminate the carbon dioxide in the blood which shows blue through the walls of the veins in typical varicose cases. Carbon dioxide is waste matter, and must be gotten rid of. Lettuce and spinach are very good here, combined, if you wish, with raw peanuts and honey. Spinach has much of the desired sodium. This will help drive out the carbon dioxide.

Varicose veins are usually found in the legs. Apply wet cloths heated to the endurance point, for one half hour. This is to bring an abundance of blood to those parts. Get into bed, lie on your back with your feet up against the wall, so that your hips will be close to the wall and the feet straight up. Grasp the ankle with both hands, as tightly as you can, and stroke the blood down the leg, thus forcing the valves to assume their normal position. Do this before you retire each evening. In the morning put on hot applications again and stroke down the blood as before. Then put on rubber stockings, which, by means of their elastic pressure, will keep the valves in their proper position throughout the day. This routine is to be repeated mornings and evenings until you have achieved your aims. Do not keep the rubber stockings on over night.

Bathe the legs in cold water every morning after the hot applications. This will contract the softer tissues of the veins. Take cold baths for the entire body also, each morning.

Q. What causes varicose veins?

A. Improper living is the cause of varicose veins as well as all other diseases. The eating of meat, dairy products, cooked foods of all kinds, condiments such as salt, the use of tobacco and alcohol—all these are man's worst enemies. And he thinks he cannot get along without them! In many instances, abnormal pressure such as that of garters, tight-fitting shoes, and the like, prevent the blood flow from taking its normal course. Heavy pressure is put upon the valves, and they collapse, at first temporarily, and later, if the obstruction continues, permanently. Women, if they must wear stockings, should wear not the round variety of garter, but a comfortable garter belt to which the stockings are fastened. Men should omit garters entirely, and both sexes should wear only shoes that permit free blood-and-air circulation.

VEGETABLE AND OLIVE OILS

Q. Please tell us how one can judge the purity of olive oil.

A. Go to see it made. Here in California there are many olive presses which you may inspect personally. The oil should be made of ripe, black olives, cold pressed. You may also judge by comparison. Have a sample of pure olive oil with you in a bottle. Compare its color with that of the oil you are thinking of buying. Another test is to boil a sample of it. If there is any fish or animal oil present, you will be able to detect it by the odor. The animal oil, too, will sputter and spit, whereas it takes a good deal of heat to make olive oil do that.

Q. Please tell what foods corn oil is best used with; also olive oil.

A. Corn oil may be used on vegetables, cereals, and also on fruits. The heavier oils in general go best with vegetables. Olive oil is included here. Nut oils, on the other hand, go well with fruits. Finer oils, like olive oil, have small molecules. These small molecules will assimilate quickly and permeate the tissues. You can use oils with practically any food, if your taste calls for it.

Q. Some people claim that olive oil is constipating. Please advise us.

A. Judge for yourself. Take a dry tube; slip it through your fingers. It will drag. Now put on a little olive oil, and it will slip quite easily. Just so when you take olive oil internally. If, however, you take only a little at a time, it will be absorbed through the various membranes and practically none will get into the intestines. If you want it to break constipation, take enough, perhaps half a cup at a time. This, of course, does not have reference to salads, but as taken alone. With salads, it has practically no effect one way or the other.

Q. Do you advise the use of cotton seed oil?

A. If you like the taste, yes. Be sure that it is pure and cold pressed. All vegetable and fruit oils, provided they are not adulterated or treated in any way, may be used.

Q. Isn't it better to eat a salad without olive oil than with it?

A. In the early months of your transition from a cooked-food diet to live foods, olive oil is useful in that it makes the vegetables more palatable. Later on, when your tastebuds have become more sensitive to the natural flavors inherent in the foods, you would do well to cut down the amount of oil used, finally omitting it entirely. Olive oil, or any other oil, is not a one hundred per cent natural food. You should always preferably eat food as Nature gives it to you. If in this form it appeals to your tastebuds, well and good.

If not, let it alone. The tastebuds are the guardians of your stomach. Observe their warnings.

VEGETABLES AND LEGUMES

Q. Is the tomato a vegetable or a fruit?

A. The tomato is an herbal fruit, like the cranberry and the banana. What is an herb? It is a plant that has a non-woody stem. Lettuce, therefore, is a simple herb; also cabbage, spinach, celery, cauliflower, mustard greens, and about three hundred other plants. An herbal fruit is what the name implies—the fruit of an herb, and as regards food value, may be expected to have the qualities inherent in both fruits and herbs. Herbs should be the staple foods of humanity, our substitute for bread. They are essential to the construction of the muscular tissues since they contain much chlorophyll protein. Which shall you eat? Ask your tastebuds. They will select the food you need most, which will also be that which tastes best to you.

Q. Some people say onions are poisonous. I can eat them every day, tops and all. Is that dangerous?

A. If you like onions, they are good for you. They are food for certain people, but merely flavoring for most others, and for the latter should be cut up and mixed with other food.

So with garlic. It is a very good disinfectant and a mild, but powerful, astringent. Eat just a little every day if you like it—if possible at night.

All vegetables should be tested by your tastebuds. They should be eaten in large or small quantities, depending on your desire and the reaction obtained. If you do not care for a certain vegetable or fruit, do not eat it.

Q. Is it a good plan to use two or three green onions for flavoring salads? Will the onions cause fermentation?

A. The onions will be good for flavor, but do not use too many. If you have difficulty with fermentation in the digestive tract due to eating onions, chop up a little parsley and add to your salad. Parsley is an antiferment. Onions in themselves have done much good. They have helped in curing certain diseases, for instance, kidney trouble, and that in about six weeks' time.

Q. How should potatoes, peas, beans, etc., be served in order to be appetizing and nourishing?

A. As for peas, eat them from the pod just as they are. Some will be sweeter and less starchy than others, so sample them well before buying. Wash your string beans, let them soak in water for an hour. Then you may eat them in their natural state or add them, cut up, to salads. If you like them flavored, soak them in pineapple juice, rhubarb juice, or lemon juice, and add a bit of honey. If no fresh fruits or green vegetables should be available, it is better to eat soaked lentils or garbanzos (chick peas), or soaked wheat germs, than to cook these starchy foods.

Potatoes should be eaten raw if you care for them at all. Some people have developed quite a liking for this otherwise unpopular root. The starches so injurious in the cooked potato are not at all so when eaten in the natural state. Shred them up with onion if you do not like them plain. Try adding rhubarb or celery juice and minced parsley. The raw potato is a purifying agent, one of the very best stomach and intestine cleansers. Do not chew too fine—swallow when still somewhat coarsely broken up. These chunks will tear off the phlegmy coating of the digestive tract bit by bit and start it on the way out. The colon and bowels of most people are encrusted with phlegm—as the hot water pipes are with calcium carbonate, sometimes to such an extent that the food can scarcely pass through, not to mention being absorbed by the villi into the bloodstream. Not until your digestive tract is clean can you commence to absorb the nourishment from natural food.

Q. Does raw rhubarb contain oxalic acid?

A. No. Oxalic acid is a mineral crystal, inorganic. No organic oxalic acid has ever been found. Many people consider raw rhubarb unfit for food. Raw rhubarb or rhubarb juice will never hurt you, since the acids, when taken into the stomach, turn into sugar as in the case of lemon.

Q. What do you think of the ice plant as food?

A. Some few plants, for instance the ice plant and New Zealand spinach, have such an affinity for salt, that, especially when grown near the ocean, will draw the salt out of the air to such an extent that in some varieties of the former salt crystals will glitter on the stems and leaves. This salt is inorganic since it has not been absorbed through the roots and assimilated by the plant. The use of these plants, then, as food, is to be condemned if they are grown near the ocean. If they are grown in a place remote from the ocean, their use is permissable.

Q. How is water removed from washed lettuce or other leaves?

A. Roll your washed leafy vegetables in a clean linen cloth, or place in a large colander or wire basket and have an electric fan blow air through it. Linen is the quickest and perhaps the best. Muslin bags are also used.

VITAMINES

Q. What is the difference between the various vitamines? Are they what you mean when you speak of the life in uncooked food?

A. The vitamines are alkalis, present often in cooked as well as uncooked foods, although not so abundantly. Some of the more delicate vitamines are often destroyed through cooking or freezing. Sunshine also forms alkalis or vitamines in the skin when exposed to the direct rays. Vitamines, however, are totally distinct from the life in uncooked foods, which is invariably completely destroyed by the application of heat. There is, however, a relationship. The vita-mine forms the capsule in which the life or "vito" is contained. "Vito" is the life itself and not the container in which it is preserved as long as the food remains in its natural form. Millions of these vitamines

probably are found in every human or food cell, so
tiny are they. The vitamine, then, is just a little larger
than the vito, and serves as a sheath and protection.
Heat bursts the container and allows the vito to escape.
It is that which you smell in the air. Cook the food,
and some of the capsules will still remain in their
deflated condition, and they will have a beneficial
influence as they are still alkalis and can still serve to
neutralize acids in the body. As noted, however, many
are destroyed. So far as the nature and function of the
vito are concerned, we do not know a great deal at
present, except that it is lighter than air, extremely
volatile, and perhaps partakes of the nature of electricity as well.

What is the difference between the various vitamines? Simply the difference between various types
of alkalis. It is a technical one and not particularly
valuable for our purposes as students of health, since
all alkalis produce a uniform effect upon the body,
varying somewhat in degree.

Q. Are certain fruits, such as seedless grapes and
small oranges, devoid of vitamines?

A. Certain fruits have more vito, and consequently
vitamines, than other fruit. Fruit grown on the sunny
side of a tree usually has more vitamines than that
grown on the shady side. Sunshine, then, is a tremendous builder of vito in the fruit or vegetable. It may
be true that certain fruits contain less as a class than
other fruits as a class, but all contain a considerable
amount.

Seedless grapes perhaps do not taste as well as other varieties, you say. It may be a matter of personal taste, or, when a preference is universally expressed for one type of fruit over another, we may safely say that we prefer the one which contains the most vito. Experimentation seems to bear this out. What we speak of as a delicious flavor is the particular combination of mineral salts found in the food, plus the vito and its encasing vitamine. Cook or freeze a fruit, the mineral content remains the same, but the vito has disappeared. The molecular structure into which the mineral salts are grouped also often changes through cooking. Thus, the difference in flavor noted between cooked and uncooked food, since they no longer are the same but different. The vito has disappeared and the chemical structure has changed. Most of the vitamines (shell of the vito), too, have been destroyed.

Q. Is there only one type of vito or are there several varieties?

A. I classify them thus: if it is the carrot you are referring to, say "carrot vito"; if it is lettuce, then "lettuce vito"; tomato, "tomato vito," and so on. All these vitos ultimately may be found to be identical, but at present that is the convenient way to distinguish between the various sources of food life.

WARTS AND CALLOUSES

Q. What is the cause of warts?

A. An excess of waste matter in the system, which then collects and forms abnormal growths known as warts. It may mean a concentration of dangerous drugs

around which abnormal cell tissue is formed to pro
tect the rest of the body. Warts, like any other disease,
is an eliminative effort by Nature.

Q. In curing warts, should some external application be used in connection with the raw food diet?

A. Wind a little cotton on a toothpick and dip into
muriatic acid. Swab the wart thoroughly. The little
lump will burn through to the quick and die. Once
dead, it will drop off. The raw food diet alone, how·
ever, will in a comparatively short time get rid of these
obnoxious growths.

Q. Is the use of the caustic pencil for removing
warty growths advisable?

A. Yes, you may use the caustic pencil. Dip it into
water and rub on wet. It will hurt you when it burns
down to the tender part. If you wish to get rid of the
growth in short order, this method is as good as any.

Q. What can I do to remove a soft warty growth
near the nose?

A. This kind of wart is called a lupus, and is easily
removed by twisting a bit to get the roots loose from
the base, and then snaring it at the surface of the skin
with a silk thread. Draw tight with a double half-
hitch to shut off the circulation of the blood. Shortly,
it will turn black and drop off. This is a somewhat
heroic measure, and should it hurt too much, put on
hot applications, which will soon relieve the pain.

Another method is to focus sunlight on it through
a reading glass, not at the point where the rays cross,

but a short distance on either side. This is to prevent too painful burning. At the point where the rays cross, you can set fire to a piece of paper. The spot of sunlight should be as large in diameter as a dime. Focus it there for about ten minutes each day. The lupus will turn black and you will be able to pick it off.

Q. What is the cause and cure for callouses on the feet?

A. The most usual cause is ill-fitting footwear, tight, and cramping the feet. The callous is a protection which Nature develops to prevent the sensitive tissue underneath from being injured too much. Natural-shaped footwear should be used exclusively, preferably with open-work top to admit air to the feet.

Those who use their feet a great deal, walking or standing many hours of the day, are apt to have callouses with almost the best of footwear. Here, however, the callouses will not be unduly annoying— usually the contrary. In such a case, you should bathe your feet night and morning in hot or cold water, preferably cold. Rub them vigorously with your hands or a coarse towel when still wet. Being a natural instrument, the hands are of course the best. Massage with a bit of olive oil. Then soak a rag in lemon juice and tie on for over night. Do this every night for a week, and your callouses will commence healing. Cutting is always dangerous and does not remove the cause.

WATER

Q. Is distilled water a natural drink?

A. The best kind of drinking water is of course spring water or rain water. Even so, you would have to select a soft-water spring or filter your rain water thoroughly. In a city, with all the smoke in the air, there is little chance of getting rain water fit to drink. Some people also object to the taste as being flat. When taken off a roof, it is often contaminated with dust and rank in flavor.

When we speak of distilled water, we mean water from which the mineral matter has been artificially removed. Such water has an affinity for the body salts. It takes calcium and other minerals from the blood-stream in order to build up its natural composition again. It is true that much water has altogether too high a percentage of mineral content and that habitual drinking of such water will lead to hardening of the arteries. City water is often contaminated with chlorine, a supposed disinfectant. Chlorine, however, is a poison, harmful to the system. Water filters may be used to take out the excess minerals mentioned above and also the chlorine. There is a type of earthenware water cooler on the market which filters the water through stones. These filters may be attached to the water tap and hence cause no trouble.

The best way to get your water is through the eating of plenty of fruits—oranges, watermelons, tomatoes, and the like. You need not separate the juice. In fact, it is better to eat the fruits in their natural state. Some people think they do not get any water unless they drink out of a glass or cup. Many fruit-arians do not drink anything from one year's end to the other, since the body does not require any moisture other than that found in their food. Exceptions are made in the case of those who are much out of doors in dry climates. If you use fruit and vegetable juices (and they are very good), you may dilute them with water so as to make them easier to digest. Drink them slowly, as it is real food you are taking into your system, and not water.

Q. Should one drink eight glasses of water a day as the medical profession advises?

A. If you feel like it, do so. When you eat cooked starches, salt, pepper, meat, etc., your system will demand water to restore the balance between moist and dry. Furthermore, the bowels will usually be clogged up, which condition calls emphatically for more moisture. But when you live on a natural diet, these considerations will be things of the past; your food will usually furnish you all the water you need. If it does not, drink as much as you desire—no more. Eating dried fruits and nuts may bring such a craving.

Q. Are mineral waters, such as those from soda and other mineral springs, beneficial in the treatment of certain diseases?

A. Inorganic minerals, such as are found in so-called mineral waters, cannot be assimilated by the human body. They may act as counter-irritants to the poisons already in your system, those responsible for your disease. Therefore, temporarily a reaction for the better may ensue. It will not, however, be a lasting one. The drinking of mineral water does not aid in the expelling of harmful material from the body; on the contrary, more will be added.

WOMEN'S DISEASES

Q. Kindly tell me what I can do to prevent menstruating twice a month. My ovaries are swollen and enlarged. I follow your diet instructions completely.

A. Take hot sitz-baths lasting half an hour. Increase the heat of the water gradually. Finally, bathe all of the body touched by the hot water with cold. This should be done for several days before the periods come on. Eat avocados, too, one each morning, at least; also tomatoes, lettuce, watercress, and mustard greens. These are all splendid for your condition. Do not bathe during the periods themselves, nor exercise strenuously. As soon as they are over, take not hot, but cold sitz-baths every night. Exercise is of great value at normal times. After the sitz-baths, bring back the circulation by exercising and rubbing.

Q. I am a woman, weight 102 pounds, age 24. About three weeks ago I caught a cold and stopped menstruating. My blood is thick. Please state cause and cure.

A. If you had always lived on natural foods you would have been normal from birth; you would never have had a menstrual period. Women menstruate only because they live so incorrectly that Nature has used this method to periodically get rid of body poisons.

If you had lived on natural foods, you would never have taken cold or become irregular. There would not have been any periods. If your blood is thick, live on natural herbs and get into the sunshine.

Q. How long will a woman have to eat raw food before she will stop menstruating?

A. Consider this: wild animals never menstruate, not even domesticated cats and dogs if they live on the foods that Nature intended for them. If they do not, they will of course suffer as do humans. All do so only because they live on dead foods. When a woman has lived normally long enough, so that her physical condition is right, she will stop this wasting of vitality.

Q. How can I heal the vagina? There is much discharge.

A. Take douches. Begin with mild lemon water and strengthen until you can take it almost clear in a little warm water. After the douche, follow with two ounces of cold water. Continue this until you get relief.

Q. Will you kindly tell me what I should do for falling of the womb?

A. First of all, live on natural food from three to six months. Then do the following: take hot sitz-baths half an hour in duration, increasing the water heat gradually. Follow by a dash of cold water. Then bend over, walk about the room on your hands and feet, bear fashion. That will tip the womb forward to where it belongs. Do this exercise as long as you can, and go to bed. Repeat the bath and exercise every night and you will soon be normal again.

Q. At the oncoming of my menstrual period my stomach becomes upset. Sometimes I suffer from severe headaches a few days after the close of the period. Is the trouble connected with my stomach?

A. The eating of meat causes severe symptoms in cooked fooders during these periods. Often the mere elimination of meat will aid considerably in these cases. With us, however, the only thing that need be said is, reduce the amount of food intake during the period. Do not eat at all if you find that that helps you. The body is often overburdened with waste material at these times and requires all the energy it can muster for the purpose of elimination.

WORRY AND FEAR

Q. What food, if any, should a person eat when worried?

A. Did you ever see a worried person who was really hungry? Hunger and worry are not compatible. When you are worried do not eat. Take long, deep breaths; drink cold water and fruit juices; bathe the head with cold water. That will soon take away your tendency to worry.

Q. What is the best thing I can do for spells of despondency and worry?

A. Get out of the rut you're in: eat live food, go on a long walk into the woods, take a sunbath, go to bed early, get up early, associate with cheerful people. It may be that you are over-worked or that you are out of a job. In either case you will be unable to maintain normal stability of mind. The work you are doing may not be congenial. Nothing is more important in mental hygiene than finding one's proper place in the world. Find out what you are best fitted for and work consistently toward it. That will replace your negative by a positive attitude.

WOUNDS AND SORES

Q. I have an old sore on my leg which has not healed for years. What shall I do for it?

A. The sore will not heal because there is no healing force in your blood. To get it, you must live on live food. If you do not sleep well—sleep is essential to recuperation—try this treatment: eat apples in the morning, lettuce at noon, turnips and onions at night. Use natural foods that will induce natural sleep. Put on hot compresses. Make a poultice of chopped parsley or spinach and put it on over the sore. This will prevent decomposition and keep "proud flesh" away. Expose to air and sunshine as much as possible. In about three to six months, the wound should be healed.

Q. Please explain the word "hemoglobin."

A. It is the element in blood that causes it to thicken when exposed to the air. If your hemoglobin is sufficient, when you cut yourself the wound will soon be closed. Lacking hemoglobin, you would keep on bleeding.

Q. What is the best way to treat a finger that has been bruised?

A. Thrust it into a bowl of hot water. Keep it there until the finger gets red; then put into cold water for a moment. Massage the injured part gently. Repeat the water-dipping and massage several times.

Q. How do you care for wounds to prevent blood poisoning?

A. If your body is clean, you will not need to worry about blood poisoning. Bring about a hyperemia in the region of the wound by hot applications. Then bathe the part in a strong lemon-juice solution. Lemon is the best possible antiseptic. Get plenty of air and sunlight on the injured spot. If possible, avoid all bandaging.

INDEX

CPSIA information can be obtained
at www.ICGtesting.com
Printed in the USA
BVHW08s0145010618
517873BV00008B/228/P